P9-CEC-211

The Two-Day Diet

The
TWO-
DAY
DIET

A Metabolic and Motivational
Approach to Rapid Weight Loss

TESSA COOPER, M.S., &
GLENN COOPER, M.D.

Random House
New York

Copyright © 1988 by Tessa Cooper, M.S., and Glenn
Cooper, M.D.

All rights reserved under International and Pan-American
Copyright Conventions. Published in the United States by
Random House, Inc., New York, and simultaneously in Can-
ada by Random House of Canada Limited, Toronto.

Library of Congress Cataloguing-in-Publication Data

Cooper, Tessa
  The two-day diet.

  Includes index.
  1. Reducing diets. I. Cooper, Glenn
II. Title.
RM222.2.C614 1989   613.2'5   88-42673
ISBN 0-394-56577-0

Book design by Charlotte Staub

Manufactured in the United States of America
98765432
First Edition

To our parents

Acknowledgments

First of all, we wish to thank all those people in America, England, and Europe who participated in the test program of the Two-Day Diet. Their feedback was invaluable in shaping the program into its final form. Gale Cooper encouraged us to pursue the project and guided us down all the right paths. Leigh Wymer provided valuable technical assistance, and Lucille Barha prepared the manuscript quickly and, with Carole Eitzen, efficiently and assisted in the test program. We especially want to acknowledge the thoughtful advice and strong support of our editor, Charlotte Mayerson. Finally, we give thanks to our professors of nutrition and medicine, who taught us the importance of treating obesity and inspired us to seek innovative ways to help our patients lose weight safely and effectively.

Contents

Introduction: Anyone Can Stay on a Diet for
Two Days xi

1. How the Two-Day Diet Came into
   Existence 3
2. The Motivational Factor—the Psychology of
   Diet Failure 10
3. The Metabolic Factor: Burning Fat Is Better
   Than Burning Muscle 18
4. Introducing the Two-Day Diet 40
5. On Days 55
6. Off Days 66
7. Making the Most of Master Menus 80
8. Two-Day Diet Recipes 109

9. The Two-Day Diet Fits Your Life-style 147

10. The Two-Day Diet Exercise Program 154

11. Special Considerations for Women and People with Medical Conditions 169

12. The Metabolic Adjustment Period—Adjusting to Your New Weight 178

13. The Maintenance Period—Maintaining Your New Weight 187

Appendix I: Determining Your Weight-Loss Goal 195

Appendix II: Two-Day Diet Menu-Planning Charts for Three Weeks 197

Subject Index 219

Recipe Index 226

Introduction:
Anyone Can Stay on a Diet for Two Days

Welcome to the world of successful dieting! You've tried so hard in the past. You've bought magazines, paperbacks, and ordered crazy things from TV ads. You've starved, binged, lost a lot, and gained it back. You've eaten grapefruits, pineapples, and powdered protein. You've gone to the drugstore to get nonprescription diet pills and come home with a bag of Halloween candy. You're beginning to believe that you're doomed to failure.

Relax. Don't worry. We're going to tell you about a new concept in dieting that combines science and psychology into a powerful program that won't let you fail. We call this program the Two-Day Diet. When you're at your weakest, the Two-Day Diet is strongest. It's like a friend giving you support and encouragement. Although the Two-Day Diet is gentle on your psyche, it's tough on your fat. You will lose weight fast—many people lose nearly a pound a day during the first two weeks. And the weight you lose will be mostly fat rather than vital muscle.

Let's repeat this message because it is important: You will be able to stay on this diet until you reach your desired weight loss, because the Two-Day Diet won't let you fail. What's more, you will be able to keep the weight off indefinitely. Think about it—your last diet!

We're going to start by telling you about ourselves, because we think that credentials are important in designing diets. Tessa Cooper is a professional nutritionist who earned a master's degree in nutrition from Tufts University in Massachusetts. She is also an exercise physiologist, with a degree from Boston Bouve College of Northeastern University. She has made a successful career of teaching people about diet and exercise. Glenn Cooper is a physician and specialist in internal medicine. He trained at Harvard and Tufts universities and has been practicing medicine for several years. We think we know what we are talking about, and we believe we have designed a diet that will work for you in a very unique way.

Why have your diets failed in the past, long before you have reached your target weight loss? Temptation. Boredom. Craving. Three gremlins pushing you away from good intentions, leaning on you until you fall off the wagon and land squarely in a chocolate cake—or bag of cookies or bucket of fried chicken. Once off the wagon, it's hard to climb back on. You eat yourself back up to your original weight, or beyond, and you're back to square one, or worse.

There is another reason you have failed in the past. Many low-calorie diets produce a profound starvation response in your body. Fat and muscle are burned as fuel sources to keep up with the energy needs of the dieter. Losing fat is obviously good, but losing muscle is undesirable. If you lose too much muscle, you feel weak and look weak. Your diet has already been making you lose your will, now you're losing your might.

If you failed in the past, forget about it. You never had the Two-Day Diet before. Ask yourself:

- Would I like to lose weight fast?

- Would I like to be motivated and excited while I diet?

- Would I like to stay strong and clearheaded while I lose weight?

- Would I like to be able to have cake, ice cream, and alcoholic beverages without going off my diet?

- Would I like a diet that gives me an incredibly wide selection of food choices, with no artificial additives?

- Would I like a diet that's easy to understand and follow?

- Would I like a diet that fits my life-style and lets me enjoy my weekends?

- Would I like to learn how to maintain my weight loss indefinitely?

If your answers are yes, your answer is the Two-Day Diet. Who is the Two-Day Diet for? It's for:

- women

- men

- people who want to lose only a few pounds

- people who want to lose a considerable amount of weight

In short, it's for you.

The story behind the Two-Day Diet is in the name. Our work with overweight people has taught us that anyone can stay on a diet for two days. After two days, people start to drop out, and after one week fewer than one in five are still successfully dieting. The Two-Day Diet short-circuits failure in a radical way: You will diet intensively for only two days at a time! The Two-Day Diet has On Days and Off Days. On Days pack the power of science. Off Days have the allure of pyschology. On Days take fat off fast. Off Days defeat temptation, boredom, and craving. Combine On Days and Off Days in the right way and you've got a revolutionary new diet program at your disposal.

Interested? Read on. A week from now, you could be up to seven pounds thinner.

The Two-Day Diet

1.

How the
Two-Day Diet
Came into Existence

Most ideas are evolutionary. They generally are not conceived full-blown without prior thought and consideration. Instead, they are based on a host of learned experiences that shape the final form of the idea. Ideas that evolve from past experiences and past ideas have the benefit of incorporating their best aspects and discarding their worst. The Two-Day Diet is evolutionary. We built on past successes and past failures to produce a program that works beautifully. This is how the idea for this diet evolved.

In the past, we were traditional prescribers of traditional diets. Well over half our patients needed to lose weight. Some had diabetes, some had high blood pressure, some had degenerative disease of their hips or knees from carrying too much weight for too many years. Others had no

medical reason for losing weight but were anxious to do so
for cosmetic reasons. Being fat was harming them psychologically, causing guilt, anxiety, and depression. As provi-
ders of health care, we tried to help our patients. The tools
at our disposal were nutritionally sound, balanced diets produced by established nutritional authorities and dissemi-
nated on printed sheets, which we gave to our patients
together with a half hour or so of general nutritional coun-
seling. Sometimes we took a detailed nutritional history to
see how much they were overeating. Often, patients swore
to us that they were not big eaters even though they were
clearly overweight. Their nutritional histories seemed to
bear this out. Foolishly, we consistently assumed they were
hiding the truth from us, covering up gallons of ice cream
and bags of potato chips. Undaunted, we chose from a range
of available diets: 800, 1000, 1200, 1400, 1600, 1800 calories, etc. Our technique for matching the diet to the pa-
tient was not exactly scientific. The thought process went
something like this: Well, he's extremely overweight, so
we'd better give him a really strict one, or She'll never stay
on a strict one, so let's give her an 1800-calorie diet since
it's better than nothing. The diets were based on the four
basic food groups and provided balanced proportions of
carbohydrates, protein, and fat. They were really very good,
healthy, prudent meal plans and we put literally hundreds
of patients on them. Do you want to know how they
worked?

To our knowledge, not a single one of our patients ever
reached his or her weight-loss goal on this kind of diet.
Most never got close.

We didn't abandon this approach easily, since we had
been taught in our training that prudent, balanced diets
that modestly restricted calories were the correct approach
to the treatment of obesity. We did a survey of our patients
and found something that disturbed us. We asked for hon-

esty and we got it. Fewer than one in five people remained on the diet past the first week. Most dropped out after only two days. Our response was to increase the supervision of these diets. We sent those patients who most needed weight loss to weekly appointments with the nutritionist, who weighed them in, reviewed their progress, and taught them over and over again how to count calories. This approach proved to be equally unsatisfactory. Some people lost a few pounds over the first couple of weeks, then leveled off and stopped losing weight. Most simply got tired of appointments and stopped coming. We were not on the right track.

We turned to behavioral approaches to obesity treatment. We reasoned that our patients were unsuccessful in their dieting efforts because they had developed unhealthy eating habits. They ate too fast, they put too much on their plate, they were conditioned to eat while they watched TV. They were failing on their diet because we were doing nothing to break their deeply ingrained bad eating habits. So we sent as many as we could to behavior-modification groups. There they learned how to monitor their eating patterns and keep records. They learned how to think "good" thoughts when they ate low-calorie foods and "disgusting" thoughts when they ate cakes and cookies. They rewarded themselves with credits toward a goal when they watched TV without nibbling, and they learned how to eat slowly.

Again, the results were dismal. To be fair, a very few patients had a satisfactory outcome, with ten to fifteen pounds of sustained weight loss. But the vast majority lost a few pounds and rapidly gained them back as they lost interest in this retraining exercise. One man told us, "Behavioral modification is turning me into a lunatic. I've got two sets of poker chips on my dresser. I have good eating behavior and I transfer a chip to the good pile. I have bad eating behavior and I transfer a chip to the bad pile. If I get all the chips in the good pile, I'm supposed to buy myself a new suit. I write notes to myself all day reminding me to transfer chips in both directions. I count the piles twice a day. I'm obsessed by them. My kid knocked the piles over the other day and I actually spanked her! I'd rather be fat."

We were in a quandary. We wanted to help our patients but we were spinning our wheels, accomplishing very little. Then we had a revelation. We discovered something called the set-point theory and suddenly our failures seemed to make sense.

The set-point theory was popularized a few years ago in a book by William Bennett and Joel Gurin called *The Dieter's Dilemma*. The authors comprehensively reviewed a large amount of research on obesity and concluded that everyone has a certain predetermined thermostat setting, or set point, that controls his or her amount of body fat. Set-point theory holds that the body has a biological drive to maintain a certain degree of fat stores and will adjust hunger, physical activity, and metabolic rate to defend against being more fat or less fat. If nonobese volunteers are deliberately over-fed, most will have a great deal of difficulty gaining twenty pounds, even by doubling or tripling their normal calorie intake for prolonged periods. Withdraw these people from the overfeeding program and they will rapidly lose their excess weight and drop back down fairly close to their original weight. These people seem to have a natural set point protecting them from becoming obese. As more calories are presented than usual, the body defends itself by decreasing hunger and increasing metabolic rate. It is difficult, though not impossible, to defeat the set point of thin people. But as soon as extra feedings stop, they quickly burn up extra fat they have accumulated and return to their normal appetite, metabolic rate, and degree of body fat.

When obese patients are placed on a calorie-restricted diet, they tend initially to lose weight rapidly. Then the rate of weight loss slows and sometimes stops completely. The natural set point of the body "protects" the dieter against losing the body fat it "thinks" it needs. The body's defense is to lower the metabolic rate, producing slower burning of calories; to raise the level of hunger; and to decrease the desire to be physically active. How diabolical! To make matters worse, as soon as the person goes off the diet, weight is rapidly regained as the set-point mechanism gears up to restore the usual amount of body fat.

Fortunately, there is a natural way to reset the set point: Regular physical activity can actually lower the body's set point. Overweight people who take up exercise become leaner, burn more calories at rest, and can lose weight without dieting. Exercise, it was argued, was a more sensible approach than dieting toward achieving weight loss. Why diet when you could reset?

We thought we had seen the light. We prescribed exercise for all our patients with weight problems. We told them that exercise was the key factor in achieving their weight-loss goals. We assured them that diet was a secondary factor. Of course they needed to "watch" what they ate and avoid high-calorie desserts and snacks. But exercise would lower set point and naturally reduce weight. We sent our patients to YMCAs, health spas, and running tracks. We had them buy jump ropes, ankle weights, and dumbbells. Then we held our breath and waited for the results.

We were disappointed. There were some very real successes in a few highly motivated, enthusiastic people, but for the great majority there was minimal weight loss or none at all. We talked to our patients to try and figure out what had gone wrong. We heard the same response over and over: Weight loss was too slow for people's expectations, a maximum of about one pound per week. If weight loss was the goal, then exercise wasn't achieving that goal fast enough. Our patients became demotivated and unwilling to keep putting in the effort necessary to see whether they would lose significant weight in the long run. They stopped jogging, though they kept wearing their running shoes.

We thought about our experience. We remained convinced that exercise had to be a critical component of a successful weight-loss plan if we wanted to achieve permanent weight-loss reduction. But we realized that a diet was also essential to promote rapid weight loss. And that diet had to deal with human nature in a way in which no diet had done before.

One day it dawned on us: We needed to work *with* human nature, not against it. To get people to stay on a diet, the diet time had to be shortened. Surely, we thought, anyone can stay on a diet for two days at a time. That was certainly the key to short-circuiting the failure of traditional diets. A period of hard work followed in which we designed a scientific plan to suit the concept. When we were finished, we were genuinely excited about the final product. We believed we had developed a plan that was completely unique and destined to be successful.

We quickly put our theory to the test. We recruited fifty overweight people, twenty-two men and twenty-eight women, into a study of the Two-Day Diet. These people had weight-loss goals ranging from ten to thirty pounds. The results delighted us and thrilled our subjects. They lost large amounts of weight easily, without unpleasant side effects. They felt alert and strong while they were losing weight—strong enough to remain very active. They also told us that this was the first diet they had ever tried that was fun to be on. They actually enjoyed dieting! And most important, forty-five of the fifty subjects achieved their target weight loss within four weeks. Many achieved it within two weeks. One woman lost twenty-five pounds in four weeks.

Before long, the Two-Day Diet was spreading by the grapevine. Our subjects were giving copies to friends and family, and we began receiving requests from people who had heard about our plan. Hundreds of people in the United States and Europe have now tried the Two-Day Diet and the numbers are growing. The feedback has been tremendous and, hence, this book. It is our hope to help you lose weight now and to show you how to keep the weight off. Motivation and metabolism are at the center of the Two-Day Diet. Before getting into the mechanics of the diet, we describe how these factors work in your body—and in your mind.

2.

The Motivational Factor—
the Psychology of Diet Failure

Most diets fail. Despite the best initial intentions, the vast majority of dieters never reach their target weight-loss goals. Many never get close. And those few who are successful often find that the pounds pile back on as soon as they go off their diet. Is the fault with the dieters or their diets? We think that the diets are to blame and firmly state:

There Is No Such Thing as a Bad Dieter, Only Bad Diets

Regina is a case in point. She is a medical secretary in her late twenties who for several years has fought the battle against fat. When Regina was in high school, her weight was stuck at 122 pounds no matter what she ate. She was

active and athletic, and despite a height of only 5'4", she
was a top player on the girl's basketball team. She showed
us a team photo from her school yearbook but had to point
herself out. She had changed so much in the past decade!
As she told it, "In school I never had to watch my weight.
I was a size eight and loved to go clothes shopping. In
secretarial school I gained a few pounds, probably because
I stopped playing sports. I wasn't too concerned at the time
because I thought it would stop there. Everything changed
when I got pregnant. I gained forty-five pounds when I was
carrying Steven and lost only twenty-five after delivery.
Over the next five years I've put on another ten pounds or
so. Now I weigh 156 and I have to wear size 14 dresses. I
hate shopping, and I am self-conscious and miserable about
my weight."

In an effort to help herself out of her predicament, Regina
became a "professional" dieter. She tried them all. She
bought every woman's magazine that had a diet article. She
devoured the best-seller list for diet books. She tried self-
help classes. She went from one diet to another and failed.
"I hate dieting, really. Dieting makes me feel deprived and
abnormal. My husband is slim so I have to serve up beau-
tiful meals for him and my son while I have horrible food.
I usually stay on a diet for only a week or so. Then I can't
stand it anymore. The most I ever lost was eight pounds,
and I always gain it back between diets."

We set Regina a reasonable weight loss goal of eighteen
pounds, to comfortably break the 140-pound barrier. She
started on the Two-Day Diet and lost six pounds the first
week, four pounds the second week, four pounds the third
week, and three pounds the fourth week. By the end of
four weeks she had lost seventeen pounds and we encouraged her to move into the maintenance phase. Six months
later, she had lost an additional two pounds and had a stable
weight of 137 pounds. She looked wonderful. She told us,

"I couldn't believe how easy it was to lose this weight. I mean it took some effort, obviously, but I always felt motivated. I knew I only had to dig in for two days at a time, and that made it different from any other plan I tried in the past. It was easy to use this diet at work in the cafeteria. I'm a size 10 or 12 now, depending on the style. I'm even shooting basketballs on the driveway with my son. It's great."

Regina and the other Two-Day Dieters succeed where other dieters fail because other diets ignore the importance of motivation. Motivation is a desire to reach a certain goal. For dieters, that goal is weight loss and all the things that go along with it—self-confidence, praise, feeling healthier, the ability to be more active. Unfortunately, just possessing the desire to lose weight is not usually enough to achieve the goal. On the road to success are many obstacles, or demotivators. Demotivators take the wind out of your sails and make you lose momentum. Most diets unwittingly create their own set of demotivators! If a diet does not help keep you motivated, that diet becomes part of the problem rather than part of the solution. Most diets fail because they ignore the fact that the very act of going on a diet is demotivating. Dieting deprives us of something we need and want—food. Food represents comfort and satisfaction. It is soothing and creates a feeling of well-being. Unless a diet can boost motivation, the only weapon against distressing feelings caused by food deprivation is the dieter's willpower. As most dieters know, willpower alone is no match against food deprivation. Let's examine the reasons why most diets fail. Think about diets you have been on in the past and see if they don't fall into one or more of these categories.

Most Diets Do Not Offer Incentives and Rewards

In a time of deprivation, it is natural to look forward to the moment when the deprivation will stop. In almost all diets, the deprivation ends only when the diet ends. That means that you have to hold on and endure all the negative aspects of a diet for weeks at a time. Some diets tell you that you can keep motivated by imagining how great you'll look in a swimsuit—in a month or so. Some counsel you to weigh yourself every day or two as an incentive to egg you on. We say that these kinds of maneuvers just don't work. Real people need real incentives and real rewards. And these rewards have to be provided regularly for meeting short-term, not long-term, goals. A weight-loss goal several weeks in the future is not a strong enough incentive to keep most people going. It is simply too easy to go off a diet. You need stronger, more immediate incentives and rewards to keep your diet moving ahead successfully.

The Two-Day Diet Offers This Powerful Incentive: Diet for Only Two Days and Reward Yourself with an Off Day

Most Diets Are Boring and Tedious

It is said that variety is the spice of life. If this is so, then many diets make life very bland indeed. We all enjoy variety in the meals we eat. If you weren't on a diet, you wouldn't dream of having similar foods on your plate day after day and week after week. Yet most diets offer few food choices. Some are ridiculously restrictive, essentially limiting you to a single food or type of food for the duration of the diet. Man should not survive on fruit alone—or rice

or powdered protein. These kinds of diets seem appealing
at first, since they are so easy to understand. But they are
not easy to follow. The dieter is soon overcome with the
monotony of it all and just gives up after a few days.

*The Two-Day Diet Offers a Virtually Unlimited Variety of
Exciting Real Foods and Gourmet Meals. You Never Have
to Eat the Same Meal Twice*

Most Diets Are Not Practical

Most popular diets insist on imposing what we call
magical meals on dieters. Magical meals are fixed menus
and meal plans. You've seen them. For lunch on Tuesday
you must have a spinach salad with chopped egg and five
crackers and one apple. For dinner on Friday it's baked
chicken, broccoli, and half a grapefruit. Why must you have
these particular meals on those particular days? It's magic.
There's really no other explanation. The authors of these
diets seem to expect you to believe that these fixed meals
are essential for the diet to succeed. The biggest problem
with magical meals is that they are very impractical. Dieters
are forced to adapt their life-style to these fixed-plan diets.
They have to take the menu plans with them to the su-
permarket to accommodate meals at home. But what about
meals at work and restaurants and dinner parties? Good
luck. Fixed meal plans have caused many a dieter to go off
his or her diet.

Other diets recognize that magical meals are unnecessary
for a successful diet, so they give people choices. Unfortunately, most of the schemes for providing choice are hope-
lessly confusing—wheels and targets and complicated lists
of exchanges. Some of these plans seem to have been cre-

ated for overweight engineers! If you have trouble understanding a diet, you will have very little chance of sticking to it.

The Two-Day Diet Is Practical, Easy to Use, and Easy to Follow. It Has a Unique Menu System That Is Straightforward and Understandable

Most Diets Don't Satisfy Your Natural Cravings

Everyone has cravings for certain foods, often sweets. Some scientists believe that there is a center in the brain that controls our cravings for sweet foods. Certain individuals tend to have stronger cravings than others, and certain foods, like chocolate, seem to be particularly addictive. Nondieters don't have to worry too much about giving in to their cravings every so often. On most diets, giving in to a natural craving is strictly forbidden. Don't touch that cake! Have a nice piece of fruit instead. Forget about blue cheese salad dressing, use lemon juice. And if you happen to like beer or a glass of wine or a cocktail, you're out of luck.

The Two-Day Diet Allows You to Satisfy Your Natural Food Cravings

Most Diets Turn You into a Guilt-Ridden Cheater

Cheating on diets is a way of life. It happens because people are, after all, human. Everyone does it, but most diet plans ignore this fact. So what are you supposed to do when you cheat? Feel guilty, of course. And each time you cheat you feel more and more worthless, until you decide that this is no way to live. Then the diet goes out the window. You've been set up to fail.

The Two-Day Diet Lets You "Cheat" on Your Favorite Foods Without Guilt

Most Diets Don't Produce Fast, Consistent Results

Diets may be categorized by the rate at which they produce weight loss. Some severely restrictive diets rely on periods of semi-starvation to promote extremely rapid weight loss. These diets are not safe unless they are conducted under intensive medical supervision. On the opposite pole are mildly restrictive diets, which undercut daily calorie needs by a small margin. These diets produce weight loss at a snail's pace. In our experience, this kind of slow weight loss is not sufficiently motivating to keep a diet moving forward to successful completion. Other diets give a good initial rate of weight loss that trails off dramatically after the first week. Interest tends to wane as weight loss slows. In order to maintain a high level of motivation and reach target goals, a dieter has to maintain a good rate of weight loss.

The Two-Day Diet Promotes Rapid, Safe Weight Loss Throughout the Entire Dieting Period

Most Diets Make You Hungry

Hunger is a major enemy of dieters. Nothing is as demotivating as a diet that produces chronic hunger, and most diets do just that. Most people can withstand hunger for just so long, especially when they have free access to a full refrigerator.

Many Two-Day Dieters Experience Less Hunger Than on Conventional Diets

Most Diets Ignore Your Life-style

Most diets seem to forget that you may have a job, that you may eat in a company cafeteria, that you may go to restaurants, that you may go to dinner parties, and that you like to enjoy your weekends. When these facts of life are ignored, a diet doesn't have much chance of success. Diets that rely on magic meals particularly ignore the realities of life. It is absolutely essential that a diet have the flexibility to accommodate people who work and socialize.

The Two-Day Diet Is Designed with Your Life-style in Mind

The Two-Day Diet deals with the motivational side of dieting like no other plan. Traditional aspects of diet failure have been tackled head-on. The plan we have developed keeps you maximally motivated every day of the diet. If the Two-Day Diet only considered the motivational factor, it would be an excellent program. As the next chapter demonstrates, it also addresses the metabolic aspect of dieting, the other essential key to successful weight loss.

3.

The Metabolic Factor:

Burning Fat Is Better Than Burning Muscle

Metabolism. The word conjures up images of chemical equations, scientists in white coats, sophisticated laboratory machines. Don't be intimidated! Metabolism is simply a general term used to describe the chemical changes that occur in the tissues of the body. Some metabolic processes involve the burning of food-derived fuels to produce the energy and heat necessary to sustain life. Others have to do with the storing of food substances in body tissues for future use as fuel. Fuel burning and fuel storage—that's really what metabolism is all about.

When your body stores more fuel than it burns, you gain weight. When it burns more fuel than it stores, you lose weight. When it burns at the same rate it stores, your weight stays even. Fuel burning and fuel storage are dynamic processes. The balance may change several times each day as you eat your meals and snacks and move about and exercise. The Two-Day Diet is designed to affect your metabolism in a very positive way, by making you a fuel burner rather than a fuel storer until you achieve your target weight loss. Then you will shift over into a state of energy equilibrium and maintain your desired weight indefinitely.

This chapter describes the metabolic events that lead to fuel storage and fuel burning and explores the influences of diet and exercise. Do you have to read it to benefit from the Two-Day Diet? No, you don't. You can skip ahead and get right into the diet plan, but we've found that people on the diet become very curious about what's going on in their body that's making them lose weight.

YOUR BODY WEIGHT

Let's say the arrow on your bathroom scale points to 150 pounds. Are you fat, thin, or just right?

There is an objective answer and a subjective answer. Objectively, nutritionists and physicians rely on certain established standards to determine if someone is excessively fat. One such standard is a table of desirable weights. You've all seen these tables: Find your height on the left-hand column, then read across the range of desirable weights for each of three frame sizes—small, medium, and large. One of our patients, Anne, is 5'5" and weighed 150 pounds. This is what the height-weight table told her:

Weight

Height	Small Frame	Medium Frame	Large Frame
5'5"	117–130	127–141	137–155

Anne is a delightful woman, but she is a denier. We knew she needed to lose weight, because she had mild high blood pressure and a family history of diabetes developing in middle age. Also, our eyes told us she was fat. However, armed with the height-weight table she was disinclined to lose weight, insisting she was a big-boned person who fell squarely in the acceptable range for the large frames.

The difficulty in judging frame size is, of course, one of the problems with standard height-weight tables. The desirable weight range for a 5'5" woman is an astonishing thirty-eight pounds from the low end of the small frame to the high end of the large frame. People tend to play the frame-size game with themselves. Deniers like Anne think they have large skeletons, while people who are overly hard on themselves assume they have small frames and huge thighs. Another problem with these standard tables is that they are very misleading if weight is composed of an unusually high proportion of muscle. Consider this professional football player who is six feet tall:

Weight

Height	Small Frame	Medium Frame	Large Frame
6'0"	149–160	157–170	164–188

He is a superbly conditioned athlete who is both strong and agile. He weighs 225 pounds. The table says he is obese. Would you want to tell him that? Obviously, better methods are needed for determining whether someone is excessively fat.

Several good methods do in fact exist, involving measurements of the total fat content of the body. The accepted standard is that a woman is obese if her body fat is greater than 30 percent of her total weight. A man is obese with body fat greater than 20 percent. In contrast, good female and male athletes generally have a fat content under 20 percent and 10 percent, respectively. Using this definition, about 25 percent of women and 12 percent of men in America are obese. That means nearly 40 million people!

One excellent method for assessing body fat involves underwater weighing. Your weight in water is determined by how much water your body displaces (remember Archimedes?). This weight is compared to your weight in air. The ratio of weight in water to weight in air allows a precise calculation of how much body fat you have. It's called hydrostatic weighing and you can't do it in your own bathtub; it takes special equipment.

With Anne, we took the unusual step of urging her to have hydrostatic weighing at a local health spa. At her next office visit, she sheepishly produced a computer printout that gave her body fat content as 35 percent. We knew it, deep down she knew it, but it took a computer to tell her she was fat.

Most people do not need height-weight tables or hydrostatic weighing to tell them if they have excessive body fat. Most people just know it subjectively—you know how you look, you know how you feel, and you know how your clothes fit. The "mirror test," for most people, works well. If, undressed and standing in front of a full-length mirror, you think you're fat, you probably are. Of course some people have psychological disorders that distort their perception of what their body looks like. These unfortunate individuals believe that they have a weight problem despite objective evidence to the contrary. Disabling eating disorders such as anorexia nervosa and bulimia may result. Most people, however, are good intuitive judges of their body-fat content and even know approximately how much weight they need to lose. You probably have a figure in mind right now. Let's say it is fifteen pounds. If your dieting goal is simply for your scale to indicate you are fifteen pounds lighter, you are not fully serving yourself. Why? Because:

All Pounds Are Not Created Equal

YOUR BODY COMPOSITION

To understand why "all pounds are not created equal" you need to understand the nature of your body composition. In essence, your body is a storage tank of energy-producing, life-sustaining fuels and water. This storage tank is divided into four major compartments: a fat compartment, a carbohydrate compartment, a protein compartment, and a water compartment. In obesity, the fat compartment is too full. The Two-Day Diet is designed to drain the fat compartment while having relatively minimal impact on the others, especially the protein compartment. We want you to lose pounds of fat, not pounds of muscle protein.

The typical American or Western European diet contains 46 percent carbohydrate, 42 percent fat, and 12 percent protein. However, the fuels we store are in entirely different proportions. Let's examine each food component and its corresponding body storage form more closely. This is the best way to understand how diets work and how the Two-Day Diet is unique.

Carbohydrate Storage

Plants make carbohydrate in the presence of sunlight, and we ingest plants and plant byproducts in the form of starches and sugars for nourishment, and cellulose for fiber. Starches are abundant in foods such as cereals, breads, potatoes, and pasta.

When we eat starches and sugars, the body digests them, or breaks them down, into the simple sugar glucose. Glucose can be used as an immediate source of energy. Each gram of carbohydrate utilized by the body produces 4 (kilo) calories of energy. The calories stored in carbohydrate are released to supply energy for the many essential needs of the body, such as heat production, muscle movement, and production of body chemicals.

Your body requires a certain number of calories each day just to meet essential needs. Eat enough to exceed these needs and fuel is stored and weight is gained. Fall short of these needs and stored body fuel is burned, producing weight loss. The daily number of calories required to break even—no weight loss, no weight gain—varies from person to person, depending on age, sex, size, genetic predisposition, and level of physical activity. The daily requirement for a typical middle-aged American man engaging in light physical activity, with no strenuous exercise, averages 2700 calories. For an American woman, that figure is 2000 calories.

What happens when you have reached your daily break-even point and you eat additional carbohydrate? The body stores the excess, in the form of glycogen, in the liver and in muscle. Though carbohydrate makes up such a large percentage of our diet, the body has a very limited capacity for storing glycogen. The combined caloric value of all the glycogen stored in the body is only about 1100 calories. This is well below your total caloric requirements for a single day. Let's say that you have stored all the glycogen you can possibly store but you go on eating carbohydrate. What happens next? Unfortunately, the body has an efficient and unlimited capacity for converting extra carbohydrates into *fat*. The liver does the work of converting glucose into substances called fatty acids, which are carried in the bloodstream to fat tissue or adipose cells for the final production of fat. Adipose cells become packed full with fat droplets. They are essentially tiny bags of grease.

Some of the Excess Carbohydrate in Your Diet Is Stored as Glycogen but Most Is Stored as Fat

Fat Storage

Some sources of fat in our diet are visible and easily identifiable: butter, margarine, salad oil, and the fat surrounding a cut of meat. Visible fat accounts for about 40 percent of the fat we eat. The rest is invisible and includes the fat marbled throughout meat, fat in egg yolks, milk, nuts, and some whole grains. In the typical Western diet about two thirds of dietary fat comes from animal sources, one third from plants, primarily as vegetable oils.

Fats, like carbohydrates, can be used as immediate sources of energy for the body. They and their derivatives are an important fuel for exercising muscles and the heart. Fat is a very concentrated source of energy. Each gram provides nine calories of energy, over two times as much energy as an equivalent amount of carbohydrate or protein.

When your daily calorie requirement has been satisfied, what happens to excess dietary fat? You guessed it: it is stored as *fat* in your body. Fat is by far the largest reservoir of body fuel. A nonobese person has about 20 percent of his or her body weight as fat stores, with a caloric value of about 140,000 calories, enough to meet minimal daily requirements for almost two months. In obese people, fat holds over 500,000 calories in storage, enough to sustain a person for at least six months. If you recall, carbohydrate storage provides an energy reserve of only 1100 calories. Why does the body use fat as its preferred storage form of energy? For various reasons, fat storage is more efficient. It is a better investment than carbohydrate storage, and the body is a smart investor. To summarize:

Excess Fat in Your Diet Is Stored as Body Fat

Protein Storage

Proteins are complex substances made up of structural building blocks called amino acids. All living tissue contains protein. The most active and abundant tissues of animals, the organs and muscles, are very high in protein content. Protein is stored in the whites of eggs, to provide for tissue growth in birds. Plants also store protein in the seed and the leaf. On a dry-weight basis, lean meat and fish are about 75 percent protein, eggs are about 50 percent protein, spinach is 40 percent protein, and soybeans are 35 percent protein.

To be absorbed, dietary proteins must be broken down in the digestive tract so they can pass into the bloodstream and be carried to the tissues. The body needs amino acids for the growth and maintenance of all body tissues—muscle, organs, bone, teeth, hair. They are also essential for formation of essential body compounds such as hormones, enzymes, and antibodies.

The major storage form of body protein is muscle tissue. A fully grown adult holds about 40,000 calories in muscle storage. However, it is very clear that muscle is not a good energy storage depot to fuel the needs of a dieter. First of all, it is not as rich a source of energy, yielding only 4 calories per gram compared to 9 calories per gram for fat. Also, muscle has important functions for strength, health, and tone, whereas excess fat is nonessential, inefficient, and generally detrimental to health.

What happens when you have taken in enough calories to meet your energy needs for the day and you eat extra protein? The answer depends largely on your degree of physical exercise. The body has little use for excess protein and actually has no place to store it. The liver removes the nitrogen portion from amino acids, and the remaining substances are converted to glucose and fatty acids. And you remember what the body does with excess glucose and excess fatty acids—it uses them to make *fat*. On the other hand, if you have been exercising your muscles, you have been stimulating them to grow larger. Muscles grow as bundles of long protein fibers that are laid down on existing muscle tissue. Children naturally form new muscle tissue as part of the overall growth process. Adults must exercise their muscles to make them larger. With exercise, some of your excess dietary protein can be used to enlarge your muscles rather than form new fat deposits. To summarize:

Excess Protein in Your Diet Is Stored as Fat but Exercise Can Favor Storage of Protein as New Muscle

What About Alcohol?

Alcohol is neither protein, carbohydrate, nor fat. It is formed when sugar is fermented by yeast enzymes. Alcohol has a greater caloric content (7 calories per gram) than carbohydrate or protein but less than fat. Therefore, alcohol is a fairly rich energy source. The body tends to burn alcohol for energy very quickly, in preference to glucose and fatty acids. Alcohol is used right away rather than stored. But whenever alcohol is burned, another energy source is not burned, leading to excess glucose and fatty acids—and storage of *fat*. To summarize:

> *Excess Alcohol in Your Diet Leads Indirectly to Storage of Fat*

The Bottom Line

When you eat more than you need to meet your daily energy needs, your body will efficiently store the excess. Excess carbohydrate, protein, fat, and alcohol are all stored as *fat*. Fat is the richest depot when energy is needed. However, protein stored as muscle is also an important and available energy source. But *all pounds are not created equal.* Excess pounds of fat are unnecessary and expendable. Pounds of muscle are vital and essential. The Two-Day Diet is designed to:

- STOP FAT STORAGE

- PROMOTE FAT BREAKDOWN

- PRESERVE VITAL MUSCLE

YOUR METABOLISM

We've seen how the food we eat is stored. Now we need to explore what happens when you no longer eat more than you need but, instead, eat less than your body needs to meet daily energy needs.

"Fed" versus Fasting

The body uses and stores food efficiently and rapidly. Within a few hours of completing a meal, excess nutrients have been packed away in glycogen and fat stores. Scientists call this postmeal period the fed state. However, metabolism is a dynamic process. The body needs a constant supply of energy to keep vital organs functioning. If dietary nutrients are not immediately available, the body switches to a fasted state. During the fasted state, energy requirements are met by burning fuel stores.

The transition from the fed state to fasted state occurs about six to twelve hours after food is eaten. This transition is tightly regulated by rising and falling levels of hormones produced by the pancreas gland. One of these hormones is insulin, the substance that many diabetics lack. Immediately following a meal, insulin is released into the bloodstream, stimulating a variety of processes designed to enhance fuel storage. Several hours after a meal, insulin levels fall, triggering processes that promote the breakdown of stored fuels.

During the day, most people take in food every four to six hours. A fed state is generally maintained provided that the calories consumed exceed the calories burned in physical activity. People will usually switch over to fasted-state metabolism during the interval between the evening meal and breakfast. During the overnight fast, the body starts to drain its storage compartments. The first compartment to be affected is the carbohydrate store, glycogen. A large proportion of available glycogen is burned overnight to meet the energy needs of the resting body. By the time you awaken in the morning, you are well into the fasted state. With breakfast, the fasted state is quickly reversed.

What would happen if you were to skip breakfast and start a total fast? Your body would react by starting to drain all its storage compartments. Glycogen stores would soon be depleted. At that point, muscle and fat stores would have to be consumed to provide life-supporting energy.

The body needs a constant supply of blood glucose to fuel the brain and other vital organs. During the fasted state, glycogen is converted to glucose. Glucose production does not cease with depletion of glycogen. Amino acids in muscle protein may also be converted into this critical fuel when energy is needed. In a total fast, muscle is rapidly broken down and burned as fuel. If a total fast were to continue for a prolonged period, loss of muscle protein would inevitably lead to serious medical complications.

Fat cannot be converted into glucose. In the fasted state fat is broken down into its components, fatty acids and glycerol. Fatty acids are a rich source of energy for all the tissues in the body. Fat is the most abundant reservoir of fuel available to the fasting individual and does not have the same important functions as muscle. Fat is expendable, muscle is not.

Dieting and the Fasted State

A diet that provides fewer calories than are needed to meet daily energy requirements and a total fast differ only in their degree of caloric deprivation. Both place the body in a fasted state. Both produce an energy deficit, with burning of fuel stores. Both cause weight loss. However, in a diet, the fasted state can be controlled. The rate of weight loss and, more importantly, the kind of weight loss can be adjusted by manipulating the amount of food and type of food consumed. In contrast, a total fast is an uncontrolled metabolic freefall that can lead to disastrous, unhealthy results.

What then is the ideal metabolic profile of a weight-reduction diet? 1) The diet should cause predictable, controlled weight loss. Results should be rapid but not precipitous. It is safer to walk down a steep slope than to step off a cliff. 2) The diet should cause fat burning in preference to protein burning. 3) The diet should curb appetite.

These metabolic effects can be achieved by deliberately *unbalancing* the usual proportions of protein, carbohydrate, and fat in the diet. An unbalanced diet? From childhood, we are taught to eat a *balanced* diet, with ample representation from all major food groups. Can an *unbalanced* diet possibly be good for you? In our opinion, the answer is yes—and no.

An Unbalanced Diet

Scientists have known for years that restricting carbohydrate foods in the diet will produce certain predictable metabolic effects that may be useful to a dieter. A host of popular diet plans have been developed that exploit the potential benefit of low-carbohydrate diets. If the level of carbohydrate is restricted in a diet, the proportions of fat or protein must necessarily be higher. Some diet plans have proposed high-fat, low-carbohydrate regimens, but increased dietary fat is medically inadvisable. The typical Western diet is already too high in fat.

Low-carbohydrate, high-protein (LCHP) diets make more sense. Carbohydrate is restricted, fat is somewhat limited, and protein is supplied in generous proportions. The total daily amount of calories must be less than daily energy needs. Otherwise you could easily gain weight on a LCHP diet: The LCHP diet induces a particular kind of fasted state. The body still reacts to a caloric deprivation by draining muscle and fat stores, but it appears to prefer

to burn fat. Diets low in carbohydrate cause less insulin to
be released from the pancreas than diets high in carbohydrate. High insulin levels signal the body to store food; low
insulin levels are a signal to burn nutrient stores. When
insulin levels are reduced, fat stores are rapidly consumed.
Evidence for rapid fat burning comes from the fact that
people on LCHP diets develop a metabolic state known as
ketosis. Ketones are metabolic byproducts of fat burning.
When fat is broken down slowly, ketones are eliminated
from the body just about as fast as they are produced.
However, with accelerated fat burning, ketones accumulate
in the blood stream and ketosis develops. Ketosis from a
LCHP diet is generally not harmful. Patients with diseases
like uncontrolled diabetes or severe alcoholism may develop
extreme degrees of ketosis that can be dangerous, but the
ketone levels in these individuals are vastly higher than in
dieters.

What happens to muscle stores on LCHP diets? There
is good scientific evidence that people who stay on LCHP
diets for prolonged periods of time preserve their muscle
mass well as they lose body fat. The short-term effect of
LCHP diets on muscle preservation has not been exten-
sively studied, but it is a reasonable assumption that even
in the early phases of LCHP diets, muscle is relatively
spared as fat is burned. During caloric deprivation, critical
levels of blood glucose are maintained by breaking down
muscle protein and converting the amino acids into glucose.
The high intake of dietary protein in LCHP diets provides
amino acids for conversion to glucose, which theoretically
reduces the need for muscle breakdown.

LCHP diets also affect the appetite. Many individuals
develop appetite suppression with the ketosis of LCHP
diets. The mechanism of this effect is unclear, but a direct
action of ketones on the appetite centers of the brain is

possible. In some people, the effect is profound and they are able to stay on severely calorie-restricted LCHP diets for months without hunger pangs.

The initial weight loss on LCHP diets can be quite rapid. In the first few days of these diets, much of the loss is water weight. The body eliminates ketones from the system by filtering them through the kidneys and passing them into the urine. Ketone elimination leads to simultaneous elimination of the mineral sodium and a great deal of water. Excessive urination is the rule during the early days of an LCHP diet. Water loss returns to normal after several days. After that, fat burning is the main factor in weight loss.

In summary, LCHP diets generally cause rapid fat burning, relative muscle preservation, appetite suppression, and quick results early on. Sounds great. What's the catch? The catch is safety.

LCHP Diets—the Margin of Safety

LCHP diets can be divided into two classes: those that provide protein in liquid form and those that offer protein in the form of real food. Some of the early liquid-protein diets available in the 1970s were, frankly, dangerous. Lacking certain essential amino acids, they created catastrophic nutritional imbalances within the body. Dozens of people died from severe irregularities of their heart rhythm. Modern formulations of liquid-protein diets usually have high-grade protein, with all essential amino acids present. The margin of safety of these formulations is undoubtedly higher than earlier products. In fact, the safety of the highest quality liquid-protein formulas is probably equivalent to real-food LCHP diets that include lean meat. Unfortunately, even modern LCHP diets that provide under 800 calories per day are still not entirely safe.

Excessive water loss during the initial stages of the diet can make people dizzy and faint. Sustained ketosis on LCHP diets can lead to a variety of imbalances of vital minerals, including potassium, sodium, chloride, calcium, and magnesium. Deficiencies of these minerals can cause fatigue, lethargy, constipation, irregular heartbeat, and other medical problems.

LCHP diets can be used safely if they are administered under close medical supervision. Periodic consultation with nutritionists and physicians, regular blood and urine tests, and careful mineral and vitamin supplementation according to results of medical tests is required to be absolutely certain that serious harm will not come to the LCHP dieter. Many communities now have private medical clinics that offer good medical supervision of low-calorie LCHP programs. However, these clinics tend to be quite expensive—two thousand dollars or more for a supervised program—and there is no guarantee that you will be able to tolerate the diet without disabling side effects. Furthermore, these diets become the dominating feature in the life of the dieter and his or her family. Constant clinic visits, odd meals, and inability to socialize properly all create substantial disturbances and conflicts. Is there a way to avoid the negative aspects of LCHP diets while preserving the positive ones?

The Two-Day Diet Is Designed to Exploit the Positive Aspects of LCHP Diets Without Subjecting the Dieter to Medical Risk, Inconvenience, or Great Expense

Metabolism and Exercise

Exercise can affect your metabolism as profoundly as diet. To ignore this effect is to ignore an important dieting tool at your disposal. Any diet plan that minimizes the role of exercise is no plan you want for yourself. Contrary to popular belief, exercise does not have to be terribly strenuous to yield substantial metabolic benefits. In fact, relatively gentle exercise can aid in fat burning and muscle preservation.

The exercising body is like a gasoline-powered machine. The longer and harder that machine must work, the more gasoline is required to keep it going. The fuel for the exercising body is stored nutrients—carbohydrate and fat. Certain activities have a greater metabolic cost than others. To pay the metabolic cost, the body must dip into fuel reserves and drain storage compartments.

Overweight people actually have an advantage when it comes to exercise. For any given activity—walking, gardening, cycling, golf—a heavier person expends more calories than a lighter person, simply because more energy is required to keep a heavier person in motion. If a 120-pound man plays golf for an hour, carrying his own bag of clubs, he will use about 278 calories. However, a 200-pound man engaged in the exact same activity will expend about 464 calories. These are approximate energy costs for various common activities for a 160-pound woman:

lying in bed	75 cal/hour
sitting/reading	77 cal/hour
bowling	218 cal/hour
golfing with power cart	224 cal/hour
slow walk (2 MPH)	224 cal/hour
raking leaves	298 cal/hour
slow swimming	307 cal/hour
brisk walk (4.5 MPH)	422 cal/hour

light aerobic dancing	432 cal/hour
bicycling	508 cal/hour
slow jogging (12 minutes per mile)	632 cal/hour

None of these activities is particularly strenuous for most healthy individuals. Yet they all burn calories and all promote weight loss. You may well ask: If light exercise is good, then isn't heavier exercise better? Heavy exercise, like running, fast cycling, intense aerobic dancing, and competitive sports, is fine for people who have worked their way into a state of good physical conditioning over a period of time, but it is terrible for someone who is overweight, out of shape, and dieting. In these individuals, heavy exercise can place great strain on muscles and joints. Athletic injuries are common. An excessive burden may also be placed on the heart. Furthermore, heavy exercise does not burn body fat as efficiently as light exercise. This is an important point:

Light Exercise Burns More Fat Than Heavy Exercise

In heavy exercise, the primary fuel to support muscle activity is the carbohydrate store, glycogen. Very little body fat is burned to support a session of heavy exercise lasting under thirty minutes. Even during prolonged heavy exercise lasting up to two hours, only fairly small amounts of fat are broken down.

The situation is quite different with light exercise. The principal fuel for muscular activity during light exercise is fatty acids from the breakdown of fat. The longer the duration of the light exercise, the greater the reliance on fat burning. More calories may be expended with heavy exercise, but proportionally more fat is burned with light exercise.

Exercise also has important effects on the lean tissue of the body. Light exercise will stimulate muscles to enlarge in individuals who have not participated in exercise programs for a while. Substantial muscle enlargement can be achieved through weight training, working muscles against a resistance with barbells or fitness machines. It may surprise you to know that weight training can produce good muscular growth even during a reduced-calorie diet provided the diet contains a moderate amount of protein. Exercise can help to preserve and indeed build muscle during a weight-reduction diet.

Muscular development is critically important for the dieter, not only for the sake of appearance and endurance but also for metabolic reasons. Muscle is the greatest consumer of energy in the body. Every pound of muscle added to your body increases the resting metabolic rate by 50 to 100 calories. If you increase your muscle mass by five pounds, you will burn up to an additional 500 calories per day at complete rest!

Many women are concerned that adding muscle will make them look masculine. This is simply not the case. Unless a woman is a dedicated body building athlete, she will not become muscle-bound. Women lack the hormones that lead to bulging muscles. Women can increase their muscle mass and still lose inches on hips, waist, legs, and arms.

It is difficult to achieve rapid, significant weight loss through exercise alone. But combine the right kind of diet program with the right kind of exercise program, and results can be spectacular. All diets, even low-carbohydrate high-protein diets, will cause some muscle to be lost, even though the primary target of the diet is depletion of fat stores. Yet caloric restriction combined with exercise can preserve muscle or even increase it. And the weight loss is faster with a combined program, and much more likely to be permanent.

The Two-Day-Diet Exercise Program Is Specially Designed to Complement the Two-Day Diet by Promoting Fat Burning and Muscle Preservation

Diet, Exercise, and Metabolism

Fat storage and fat burning are dynamic processes. Fat stores are continuously burned to support the needs of the body and then replenished. Despite the dynamic nature of energy burning and energy ingestion most people, fat or thin, remain at roughly the same weight for long periods of time. In other words, most people are in the state of energy equilibrium. The equilibrium point, or set point, for fat people favors a high body-fat content; for thin people, it favors a low body-fat content. What are the factors that cause this difference? In other words, why do some people become fat while others do not?

New scientific evidence strongly suggests that most fat people do not eat significantly more than thin people. Rather, they tend to have lower resting metabolic rates. Since they burn fewer calories at rest every day, fat storage is favored. Furthermore, obese parents may pass on the tendency for low metabolic rates to their offspring.

Another important factor is the level of physical activity. Recently, researchers in England followed the energy intake and energy expenditure of infants born to fat and lean mothers and discovered some surprising results. Babies born to obese mothers were far more likely to become fat by the age of one year. And babies who were eventually to become fat had identical food intake and burned the same amount of energy at rest as babies who would remain lean. They burned fewer calories only because they were *less physically active* than other babies. The implication of this finding is that people may inherit traits favoring activity or inactivity. Could a sedentary life-style have a genetic basis? Is being a couch potato a biological tendency rather than a state of mind?

The answer to this tantalizing question is far from certain, but it is clear that obesity in many individuals is not a primary disorder of overeating; rather, it is one of under-burning. You can perhaps take comfort in the fact that you may not be a gluttonous person and that it is your metab-olism, or your parents' metabolism, that is to blame. Un-fortunately, that knowledge alone will do little to help you lose weight. You may not have overeaten yourself into your overweight condition, but you will have to cut your food consumption and increase your physical-activity level to get yourself out of it.

And there is one more factor working against you as you attempt to lose weight. Your body doesn't really "want" you to become thinner. Anyone who has been on a diet for several weeks knows that the rate of weight loss will decline with time. Further progress eventually becomes painfully slow or grinds to a halt. An individual on a calorie-restricted diet naturally undergoes changes in his or her resting meta-bolic rate and level of physical activity. The metabolic rate falls by up to 30 percent in long-term dieters. And activity levels also fall dramatically. The end result of a decline in both metabolic rate and level of activity is diminished weight loss. The explanation for this frustrating phenom-enon is probably evolutionary. In times of famine, it is advantageous for an animal to adapt to unfavorable envi-ronmental conditions by slowing down all metabolic pro-cesses and expending less energy. In this way, fuel stores are drained as slowly as possible and survival is prolonged.

When you go on a diet, your body doesn't know or care that you are trying to do it a favor. Instead, famine-protecting metabolic processes become operative and thwart your best efforts. As far as we know, there is only one way to get over this evolutionary hurdle and continue a satisfactory degree of weight loss beyond the third or fourth week of a diet: exercise. Exercise programs can actually increase the metabolic rate by increasing the amount of metabolically active lean muscle as well as other mechanisms. If you start the Two-Day Diet exercise program when you start the Two-Day Diet, you can continue to lose pounds of fat, not muscle, at a rate that will please you and keep you motivated until you reach your target weight-loss goal.

4.

Introducing the Two-Day Diet

You are about to start a diet that is different from any other diet you may have tried in the past. Most diets require you to have superhuman willpower and to bravely suffer through day after day of deprivation. Most diets severely limit your food choices. Most diets that offer quick weight loss cause potentially damaging imbalances within your body. Many diets rely on tedious calorie counting or confusing substitution lists. The Two-Day Diet is a refreshing, innovative alternative designed to meet the needs of real people who want to lose weight rapidly without enduring psychological and physiological hardship.

Men and women like you have lost weight and have kept it off using the Two-Day Diet. Here are just a few examples of the kind of results that people have achieved.

Barbara is a fifty-nine-year-old school teacher who is 5'4" and weighed 154 pounds. Her previous best effort at dieting was a disappointment to her—seven pounds in six weeks. At the start of the Two-Day Diet, her weight-loss goal was twenty-four pounds. During the first week of the Two-Day Diet, Barbara lost seven pounds. Over the next four weeks, she lost an additional eighteen pounds and her weight was down to 129 pounds. She achieved her target weight loss and felt healthy and satisfied in the process.

Craig is a thirty-three-year-old industrial chemist who had gotten paunchy through inactivity. He is 6'1" and weighed 204 pounds. He wanted to lose fifteen pounds quickly and get back into a regular exercise program. He began the Two-Day Diet and lost fourteen pounds in fourteen days. He couldn't believe how easy it was to stay on the diet despite cafeteria lunches and business dinners.

Sandra and Howard are a married couple in their mid-forties. They are both excellent cooks and love preparing gourmet dishes for each other. However, they do not enjoy being overweight, and they felt they needed to lose fifteen to twenty pounds each. They began the Two-Day Diet together and had excellent results. Howard lost nine pounds in the first week and Sandra lost eight pounds. They both lost another ten pounds over the next two weeks, for a grand total of nineteen and eighteen pounds respectively, in three weeks. We have had several couples participate in the Two-Day Diet—husbands and wives, mothers and daughters, roommates—and have consistently noted highly favorable outcomes. Dieting with a partner is a particularly enjoyable and effective approach.

People lose weight at different rates, depending on factors such as age, sex, initial body weight, and level of physical activity. On average, people participating in our initial test of the Two-Day Diet lost six pounds during the first week, four pounds during the second week, three pounds during the third week, and three pounds during the fourth week. That means if you have an average response to the Two-Day Diet, you could weigh about sixteen pounds less four weeks from now. If you respond particularly well, your weight loss could be closer to twenty-five pounds. Men, particularly those with large frames, usually lost more weight more quickly than women. A weight loss of about sixteen pounds within three weeks was often seen in large men.

Achieving your target weight-loss goal will be cause for celebration, but that is not the final goal of the Two-Day Diet. The Two-Day Diet is designed to prevent weight regain and to ensure that your desired weight is maintained permanently. The Two-Day Diet is a comprehensive program with three phases. During the initial phase, generally lasting two to six weeks, you will lose pounds quickly and safely until you reach your desired weight. The second phase, lasting two weeks, is a metabolic adjustment period that guarantees avoidance of the rapid weight gain that many people experience when coming off a diet. Finally, the third phase teaches you how to maintain your new weight into the future. The new, thinner you will be able to reach a state of energy equilibrium, where the food you eat is well balanced with the energy you expend through physical activity.

Before starting the Two-Day Diet, you must establish your personal weight-loss goal. Most people know by intuition approximately how much weight they need to lose. It is important that you set yourself a realistic, achievable target. If you are a forty-eight-year-old woman who weighs 168 pounds, a final weight of 105 pounds is not very realistic, even if that was your weight during the Eisenhower administration. Don't set yourself up to fail. If you need to lose a large amount of weight, you can set your target in stages. Lose twenty pounds first, then see how you look and feel. You may carry on and continue to lose more weight, or you may elect to stabilize and maintain that weight for a while before attempting further weight loss.

On the other hand, if you need to lose less than twenty pounds, stay on the Two-Day Diet until you achieve this goal, then enter the adjustment and maintenance phases. If you don't trust your intuition (or the opinion of others) and want a more accurate idea of how much weight you should lose, we have provided a chart in Appendix I that lets you determine how much weight loss is needed to move you into the acceptable weight category.

Before you start this program, please heed this note of caution. The Two-Day Diet is ideally suited for most people, but *certain individuals should not participate in any diet that produces rapid weight loss.* Pregnant women, mothers who are breast-feeding, children, and teenagers should not use the Two-Day Diet. Men and women who take prescription medications should check with their physician on the advisability of a rapid weight-loss program. This is particularly important if you have diabetes, high blood pressure, heart disease, or a history of kidney problems or gout. Medical clearance is also necessary if your doctor already has you on a diet to correct a medical problem such as diabetes or high blood pressure, even if you are not taking prescription drugs. Your doctor may well advise that weight loss is precisely what you need to improve the underlying medical condition, but it may be necessary to modify the doses of your medications as you lose weight. Chapter 11, "Special Considerations for Women and People with Medical Conditions," expands on these points and will help you get the maximum benefit from the Two-Day Diet.

THE TWO-DAY DIET EXPLAINED

Motivational and metabolic concepts exist side by side in the Two-Day Diet. Taken alone, the motivational component and the metabolic component would each represent powerful dieting tools. Combined, they produce a uniquely effective and safe program.

Our work has shown us that virtually anyone can stay on a diet for two days. That two-day interval is the cornerstone of the Two-Day Diet: Diet intensively for two days with a metabolically active plan, and reward yourself with a one- or two-day interval of increased food content and choice. The Two-Day Diet divides the week into On Days and Off Days.

Monday – On Day
Tuesday – On Day
Wednesday – Off Day
Thursday – On Day
Friday – On Day
Saturday – Off Day
Sunday – Off Day

Weight loss is greatest on the two On Days. Waiting for you midweek is an Off Day, a strong incentive that makes it easy to keep going and keep losing weight. Off Days are like a carrot-on-a-stick for Two-Day Dieters. They are satisfying and rewarding but keep the diet moving ahead on track. Then use two more On Days at the end of the week and you have made it to the weekend and two full Off Days! The weekly cycle is repeated until you have reached your target weight-loss goal.

The pattern of On Days alternating with Off Days gives the Two-Day Diet something we call a motivational rhythm. When we question our dieters, they usually indicate that the rhythm of On Days and Off Days is their favorite aspect of the Two-Day Diet. Gone are the boredom and monotony of grinding out day after day of hard dieting. Gone is the feeling that time is standing still as you try to lose weight. Instead, dieting actually becomes fun! Two days of intensive dieting poses little problem when mid-week and weekend Off Days beckon. In fact, many people look forward to returning to On Days after the weekend since the rapid weight loss of On Days is motivational in and of itself. Also, the appeal of the motivational rhythm does not wear thin after a short period of time. Most people enjoy successive weeks of the Two-Day Diet as much as the first.

At this point, we want to introduce you to the concept of On Days and Off Days in greater detail, then provide you with general information about other aspects of the Two-Day Diet. The chapters that follow provide all the material you need to start the diet and follow through to a successful conclusion.

On Days

On Days provide the exact combinations of protein, carbohydrate, and fat to maximize fat burning. On Days are high in protein, relatively low in carbohydrate, and contain a prudent amount of fat. The total daily caloric content is variable, depending on personal food choices, but it ranges from approximately 700 to 900 calories. Men and women use identical menu plans on On Days for breakfasts, lunches, and dinners. A wide variety of unlimited foods with negligible caloric content are available throughout the day.

Since On Days are low in carbohydrate and high in protein, you will recognize that they are similar to the LCHP diets described in the previous chapter. Therefore, On Days promote rapid fat burning and produce a state of mild ketosis. We have found that most people on the Two-Day Diet develop a mild ketosis within twenty-four hours of beginning an On Day. Appetite suppression usually accompanies the development of the ketotic state. Hunger is generally blunted during the latter half of the first On Day and the entire second On Day. As with any LCHP diet, water loss is fairly brisk on On Days, especially right at the start of the Two-Day Diet. Generous fluid intake is encouraged during On Days to compensate for these losses. A multivitamin/mineral supplement is recommended to ensure a full complement of vitamins and minerals while calories are restricted.

On Days provide the metabolic benefits of LCHP diets, namely rapid fat burning, rapid weight loss, and appetite suppression, without the risks that may be associated with their use. After only two days, the metabolic effects of On Days are quickly reversed by an Off Day. Prolonged or severe metabolic imbalances do not occur on the Two-Day Diet.

Off Days

Off Days offer a balanced proportion of food constituents. Off Days are higher in carbohydrate and lower in protein than On Days. Fat content remains at a similarly prudent low level. Off Days do not cause ketosis, and as we have said, they reverse the metabolic effects of On Days. Off Days give substantially more calories than On Days. Women receive approximately 1200 calories per day; men receive approximately 1500 calories. This higher caloric content means substantially more food. The step-up in meal size from an On Day to an Off Day is considerable and highly noticeable. In making the transition to Off Days, most people believe they are no longer dieting. This is not the case. Off Days are sufficiently low in calories to keep the diet progressing and to ensure continuing fat loss. Nevertheless, weight loss during Off Days is slower than on On Days, due to milder calorie restriction and some regain of water weight. Off Days are intentionally designed to be gentler on your body and your psyche.

The motivational attraction of Off Days is strong indeed. Imagine feeling like you're not dieting when you really are! The impression of being off a diet is enhanced by the availability of foods we call cravers during Off Days. Cravers are the foods and drinks you especially love and the ones that are banned from most diets. Make a mental list right now of the foods you crave the most. We guarantee you most of them are available on Off Days. And you are permitted two of them per day—as desserts, as between-meal snacks—whenever you like. As with On Days, a variety of unlimited foods are also available ad lib throughout the day.

Off Days are there when you really need them—in the middle of the week and on weekends. Two Off Days over the weekend are just reward for a hard week of work. Enjoy the increased flexibility and choice over the weekend as you eat out and socialize. By Monday you will be ready and eager to resume On Days.

Master Menus

We have designed a unique method for choosing your meals for On Days and Off Days. It is a method that is easy to follow and gives a remarkable degree of diversity in meal selection. The basic instrument for meal selection in the Two-Day Diet is called the Master Menu. On Days and Off Days each have two Master Menus, one for breakfasts and one for lunches and dinners. Master Menus utilize the Chinese-restaurant-menu approach. Food choices are arranged in three or four columns, and a meal is made by choosing one from column A, one from column B, one from column C, etc. Each column contains foods with similar caloric and nutritional content. Choice is based entirely on your preference. What could be easier?

There is no calorie counting on the Two-Day Diet. Don't bother to look for calorie charts because you won't find them. We have done all the work for you. All you need to do is choose the foods and meals you like. The choice available to you is enormous—literally, thousands of menu possibilities. Or you may choose not to choose. Some people prefer repetition; for example, a similar breakfast and lunch every day. The Two-Day Diet accommodates diversity or repetition. It's your choice. Master Menus also have the built-in flexibility to easily handle cafeteria and restaurant dining. You won't have to go off your diet because you're going out to eat.

Recipes

The Two-Day Diet gives you yet another level of choice. We have created special recipes for On Days and Off Days that may be used together with the Master Menus. These recipes are quick, simple to prepare, and suitable for family meals, even if there is only one dieter in the group.

Preparing to Start the Two-Day Diet

Before you start the Two-Day Diet, read through the rest of the book so you have a clear idea of how it works and where you are heading. Grocery shopping for the Two-Day Diet poses no special problems or demands. The emphasis should be on high-quality vegetables, fruits, meats, poultry, and fish. In our opinion, quality ingredients are well worth any additional cost. When food tastes better, it is naturally more satisfying and portion size becomes less important. Certain cooking techniques enhance the natural flavors and textures of foods while limiting additional calories. These are the techniques we encourage in the Two-Day Diet. We discuss them in Chapter 7, "Making the Most of the Master Menus."

Menu planning for the Two-Day Diet is easy. You can make your choices on the spot as you go through the cafeteria line or browse through your refrigerator, or you can plan ahead and compose menus. We have provided you with some menu-planning aids. In Chapter 7, there are three weeks of sample menus for the Two-Day Diet. These sample menus demonstrate how you can use Master Menus and Two-Day Diet recipes to create interesting and appealing meals. Use these sample menus to stimulate your own ideas, or follow them to the letter if you like. The other aids for menu planning are On and Off Day blank menu charts located in Appendix II. There are enough for three weeks of planning. Some people find it easier to compose menus in advance and record them so they can recall particularly good meal plans.

There are a few simple but important rules for starting and following the Two-Day Diet.

1. For best results, start the Two-Day Diet on a Monday. This allows you to get properly into the rhythm of On and Off Days.

2. Eat *all* the food permitted during On Days and Off Days. If you eat less, you will defeat some of the important metabolic and motivational features of the

Two-Day Diet and you will be less likely to reach your
target weight-loss goal. Don't deprive yourself of cravers on Off Days. Also, don't carry over food from one
day to another.

3. Follow the On Day and Off Day schedule exactly as
   presented. *Never* use On Days for more than two days
   at a time.

4. If you go off the diet for one or more days for any
   reason, resume the sequence normally. For example,
   if you miss a Tuesday and a Wednesday, resume the
   diet on Thursday with an On Day.

5. If you develop an illness like a cold or flu or if you
   injure yourself, do not use On Days. During illness and
   injury, you need more nutrient calories to help your
   body heal and repair. Use Off Days instead, then resume the normal sequence when you have recovered.

6. Ask your pharmacist or doctor to recommend a high-
   quality multivitamin/mineral supplement and take one
   every day during the Two-Day Diet.

7. Women should frequently choose dairy foods, which
   are high in calcium. A calcium supplement for women
   may be advisable. We discuss this point more fully in
   Chapter 11.

8. Fruits and vegetables, natural sources of fiber, are important components of the Two-Day Diet. Extra fiber
   can be introduced in Off Days breakfasts in the form
   of high-bran cereals.

9. Pay attention to cholesterol. Eggs and red meat are
   available as choices during On Days and Off Days, but
   many people should limit their intake of high-
   cholesterol foods. It is prudent to have no more than
   three eggs per week.

10. Start the Two-Day Diet Exercise plan at the same time you start the Two-Day Diet.

11. Weigh yourself before you start the Two-Day Diet, then once a week on the same scale at the same time of day. Keep a record of the results.

Portion Sizes

Determining portion size is straightforward on the Two-Day Diet. All you need is a measuring cup. A food scale is useful if you have one, but not essential. Most vegetables and fruits, juices, cereals, and dairy products are measured in cups. Meat, poultry, fish, and hard cheeses are measured in ounces.

Estimating the weight of solid foods gives people the most problems. If you have a scale, use it by all means, but don't go out and buy one just for the sake of the diet. For many foods, your grocer or butcher will have done some of the work for you by noting the weight on the packet. The weight of boneless cuts of meat and poultry and lean cuts of meat will be accurate. In these cases, the purchased portion can often be divided into halves or thirds to obtain the correct portion size for On and Off Days.

The weights given in the Master Menus are cooked weights unless otherwise specified. As a rule of thumb, a portion of meat, poultry, or fish will lose 1 ounce of weight during cooking. Therefore 7 ounces of uncooked steak will yield 6 ounces of cooked meat. Since cold cuts are already cooked, their weight can be used as is.

The Two-Day Diet uses portion sizes of 4 or 6 ounces for poultry and fish and 3 or 4 ounces for meat. The following guidelines may be useful in determining portion sizes for some of the more difficult-to-gauge items.

Poultry: 4 ounces of chicken = 1 thigh plus 1 drumstick

6 ounces of chicken = ½ breast or 2 thighs plus 1 drumstick

Fish: 4 ounces flounder fillet = 2 fillets—6 inches long, 2½ inches wide, ¼ inch thick

6 ounces flounder fillet = 3 fillets—6 inches long, 2½ inches wide, ¼ inch thick

4 ounces swordfish = 3 inches long, 3 inches wide, ½ inch thick

6 ounces swordfish = 4½ inches long, 3 inches wide, ½ inch thick

4 ounces shrimp = about 8 large shrimps

6 ounces shrimp = about 12 large shrimps

4 ounces scallops = about 8 sea scallops

6 ounces scallops = about 12 sea scallops

4 ounces lobster = meat from a 1-pound lobster

6 ounces lobster = meat from a 1½-pound lobster

Meat: 3 ounces hamburger = ½ inch thick, 3-inch-diameter patty

4 ounces hamburger = ¾ inch thick, 3-inch-diameter patty

3 ounces chops (lean meat) = 1 medium chop (6–8 ounces)

4 ounces chops (lean meat) = 1 large chop (8–10 ounces)

The Two-Day Diet Exercise Plan

Before we get into the actual details of the diet, it's important to stress the necessity of combining exercise with diet. The cornerstone of the Two-Day Diet exercise plan is the concept of frequent low-intensity, or light, exercise (page 154). Low-intensity exercise is gentle on the body and does not put great strain on the heart or joints, but it is the most effective kind of exercise for burning fat. It is also very useful in preserving or even building muscle. We offer a wide variety of indoor and outdoor activities that are also enjoyable. Even if you haven't done anything more vigorous in the past year than getting up from the couch to uncork a bottle of wine, you will have no problem getting into this activity program. The adage "no pain, no gain" does not apply here. The Two-Day Diet exercise plan is painless but still gives you tremendous benefits. During On Days and Off Days you will engage in light exercise for about thirty minutes. You can do it in your living room watching TV or outdoors with your stereo headphones, at your office, or in a fitness club. You can do it any time of day—whatever suits your needs, whatever suits your schedule.

When you reach your target weight loss, you will enter the second phase of the Two-Day Diet, the metabolic adjustment period. Exercise will have helped you get there and exercise will help to keep you there. The intensity of exercise increases during the adjustment period. By this time you will be lighter and fitter than you have been in years. Two weeks later you will be into the maintenance phase where activity sessions are shorter and less frequent, but there is a good chance you will find regular exercise so invigorating you will want to keep it in your life.

The Metabolic Adjustment Period

Losing weight is easier than preventing weight regain after the diet ends. For this reason the metabolic adjustment period, the second phase of the Two-Day Diet, is critically important to your long-term success. This carefully designed two-week diet and exercise program will prevent weight regain by combating a metabolic condition known as the repletion reaction.

The Maintenance Period

When you start a diet your main concern is getting the weight off, not keeping it off. Soon you will reach the day when you have achieved your goal and need a strategy for maintaining your weight into the future. The Two-Day Diet maintenance program is sophisticated yet simple. It is based on state-of-the-art principles of nutrition and fitness. The Two-Day Diet could be the last diet you ever require.

5.

On Days

Mondays, Tuesdays, Thursdays, and Fridays are On Days. These are the days you will make the most progress in losing weight and draining your fat stores.

Men and women follow the same Master Menus for On Days. There is one Master Menu for breakfasts and one for lunches as well as dinners. A variety of unlimited foods may be used to supplement and complement the Master Menus as desired. At this time, browse through the On Days Master Menus and Unlimited Foods list to get an idea of their format. We will take you through each chart to make sure you thoroughly understand it.

ON DAYS MASTER MENU
For Men and Women

Breakfast (choose one from each column)

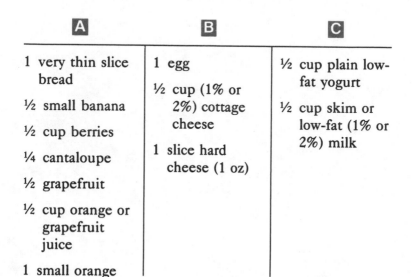

A	B	C
1 very thin slice bread	1 egg	½ cup plain low-fat yogurt
½ small banana	½ cup (1% or 2%) cottage cheese	½ cup skim or low-fat (1% or 2%) milk
½ cup berries	1 slice hard cheese (1 oz)	
¼ cantaloupe		
½ grapefruit		
½ cup orange or grapefruit juice		
1 small orange		

ON DAYS MASTER MENU
For Men and Women

Lunch/Dinner (choose one from each column)

A	B	C
1 cup asparagus spears	4–6 oz chicken	1 very thin slice bread
1 cup sliced green or wax beans	4–6 oz turkey	½ cup skim or low-fat (1% or 2%) milk
2 cups bean sprouts	4 oz lean beef, pork, lamb, or veal	1 small apple
½ cup sliced beets	4–6 oz fish or shellfish	2 apricots
1 cup chopped broccoli	½–1 (6½ oz can) tuna in water	½ small banana
6 brussels sprouts	1–1½ cups (1% or 2%) cottage cheese	½ cup berries
2 cups chopped cabbage	1 hard-boiled egg plus 1 oz hard cheese plus 1 oz turkey or ham	¼ cantaloupe
½ cup sliced carrots		½ cup cherries
2 cups chopped cauliflower		½ cup grapes
1 cup diced egglant		½ grapefruit
		1 cup diced melon
		1 nectarine
		1 small orange
		½ cup diced papaya

(continued on following page)

ON DAYS MASTER MENU
For Men and Women (continued)

Lunch/Dinner (choose one from each column)

A	B	C
1 cup diced green pepper		1 medium peach
1 cup sliced mushrooms		½ medium pear
½ cup chopped onion		2 plums
1 cup cooked spinach		⅓ cup diced pineapple
1 cup sliced summer or zucchini squash		¾ cup tomato or vegetable juice
2 medium tomatoes		

Unlimited foods such as lettuce, salad greens, and raw spinach may be added as desired. Refer to Unlimited chart.

Unlimited Foods *(use as desired during On Days and Off Days)*

---

lettuce or other salad greens
raw spinach
radishes
cucumber
celery
pickles (unsweetened)
horseradish
garlic
vinegar
diet Jell-O
mustard
soy sauce

diet sodas
club soda
mineral water
black coffee
tea, herbal tea
saccharin/
  NutraSweet
bouillon, clear broth
lemon or lime juice
salt (in moderation)
pepper
herbs
spices

BREAKFASTS

The Master Menu for breakfasts has three columns. Your meal is assembled by choosing one selection from column A, one from column B, and one from column C. Column A selections include fruit, fruit juices, and bread. Each item has a similar caloric value and content of protein, carbohydrate, and fat. You will notice that columns in Master Menus are not arranged by traditional food groups—fruits, vegetables, meat, dairy. Instead, they have been designed to facilitate creative, convenient, and practical meal planning.

Since On Days are low in carbohydrates, breads, grains, fruits, and cereals are somewhat restricted but by no means eliminated. If you choose bread for your Column A selection, it must be very thinly sliced or a low-calorie bread. Each piece should have has about 40 calories. If you cannot find this kind of bread in your grocery store, you can simply use one half slice of conventionally sliced bread instead. However, a whole slice of bread is psychologically more satisfying than a half a slice, so we prefer the very thin variety. Different types of berries—strawberries, raspberries, blueberries, etc.—are interchangeable. If you make this selection, you can have the berries on their own or mix them with the yogurt in column C. Unused portions of bananas, cantaloupe, or grapefruit can be saved in plastic wrap for another meal.

Column B entries are high in protein—eggs, cottage cheese, and hard cheese. Eggs may be prepared any style you like. If you like them fried, you can get excellent results without oil if you use a good nonstick pan. Otherwise, eggs can be boiled, poached, or scrambled without fat. Cottage cheese is available with varying percentages of milk fat. We use 1% or 2% cottage cheese on the Two-Day Diet because it is lower in calories than regular cottage cheese but has equivalent amounts of proteins and calcium. All hard cheeses like cheddar, Swiss, and American cheese are interchangeable on the Two-Day Diet. The weight of a block of hard cheese is usually indicated on the package, so a 1-ounce portion can be gauged. One conventional slice of American cheese weighs 1 ounce.

Column C choices are also fairly high in protein and are excellent sources of calcium. Your options are low-fat yogurt or skim or low-fat milk (1% or 2%). Again, higher fat varieties of dairy products only add unneeded calories.

Lunches/Dinners

A single Master Menu with three columns is used for lunches *and* dinners. A lunch or dinner is made by choosing one selection from column A, one from column B, and one from column C. Column A foods are vegetables. Measurements are primarily in cups, and unless specified, all portion sizes refer to either cooked or raw produce. Spinach is the notable exception. Raw spinach is on the Unlimited list since it is so low in calories. However, 10 ounces of raw spinach reduces to 1 cup when cooked, yielding enough calories to be included in column A. Many people prefer to use raw vegetables for lunch and cooked vegetables for dinner but it's purely a matter of preference. Large luncheon salads are popular on the Two-Day Diet. Use raw vegetables from column A, lettuce, salad greens, or raw spinach from the Unlimited list, and perhaps a choice from column B. You don't have to limit your salads to a single column A vegetable. Two or more may be combined as long as the portion size of each is reduced appropriately. For example, if you want to use tomatoes and onions in the salad, use one medium tomato instead of two, and ¼ cup chopped onion instead of ½ cup. If you desire cooked vegetables, the most nutritional and flavorful way of preparing them is steaming (see page 81). After fresh, frozen vegetables have the highest nutritional value and also are preferable to canned vegetables in flavor and texture.

Column B foods are the main course of the meal. You can choose from generous portions of poultry, meats, fish, shellfish, and cheese. You are allowed larger amounts of poultry and fish than meat because meat has a higher caloric density due to higher fat content. You will notice that there is a range of portion sizes for some of the foods: for example, 4–6 ounces of chicken, ½–1 can of tuna, 1–1½ cups of cottage cheese. You are permitted to go up to the top of the range for any selection, and most people elect to do just that. However, some people, particularly women, find that 6-ounce portions of poultry or fish, a whole can of tuna fish, or 1½ cups of cottage cheese is a larger serving than they desire. For these individuals smaller servings, down to the lower limit of the range, are allowed. Column B choices that are consistently in the low end of the range will give On Days a calorie value of about 700 calories. Consistent high-range choices will yield about 900 calories per day. Large-frame men should generally use the highest available portion sizes, but other people can make their choice according to personal preference. The Two-Day Diet is not a strict calorie-counting diet, and the total caloric content of On Days (as well as Off Days) will vary slightly from day to day depending on meal selections. There is no reason for any diet to strive for a precise, predetermined caloric level. The Master Menus have built-in flexibility and will keep you in the optimal range for fast, safe weight loss.

Techniques to prepare poultry, meat, and fish can be found in Chapter 7 (page 80). Broiling, grilling, and baking are generally the preferred methods. Cooking styles that rely on large amounts of oil and fat add unnecessary calories and, in our opinion, detract from the natural flavor of the foods. Cold cuts are popular for lunches and often used in chef's salads and/or open-face sandwiches. The last entry in column B is a combination of hard-boiled egg, cheese, turkey, or ham that is ideal for chef's salads. Canned tuna packed in water is a luncheon favorite. Tuna in oil has almost *double* the calories and should be avoided. Hot entrees are generally prepared for dinner. The large portion sizes allow for very generous and satisfying dinners.

Column C foods consist of bread, milk, and a wide variety of fruits. The availability of bread makes it possible to have open-face sandwiches. A glass of cold low-fat milk gives women another opportunity to boost dietary calcium. A selection of fruit is a good way to end an On Day lunch or dinner. Fruit is naturally sweet and can satisfy dessert cravings. If you want to use canned fruits, make sure you buy unsweetened varieties.

Unlimited Foods

Unlimited foods are an integral part of the Two-Day Diet. They provide extra content and extra flavor to meals without adding many extra calories. The basic salad fixings are all present—lettuce, salad greens, spinach, radishes, cucumber, celery. Just add column A selections and a low-calorie dressing for a fine salad. There are a variety of good low-calorie dressings commercially available, and many cafeteria and restaurant salad bars include a low-calorie choice. The calorie content of commercial diet dressings varies widely. Use those with fewer than 10 calories per tablespoon and add up to two tablespoons of dressing to each salad. As an alternative, you might like to use the recipes for low-calorie dressings in Chapter 8. One of them, a "vin-

egarette," is made exclusively from ingredients on the Unlimited list, so you can use as much as you like. Or you
can simply sprinkle your salad with freshly squeezed lemon
juice and perhaps a few turns of fresh crushed pepper.

Condiments such as unsweetened pickle, horseradish,
mustard, and soy sauce may be used freely. Ketchup is high
in calories and is therefore not an unlimited food. The sky
is the limit with herbs and spices. They add zest and sparkle
to recipes (see Chapter 7). During the first phase of the
Two-Day Diet, salt should be used in moderation but not
severely restricted. During On Days you tend to lose sodium from your body, and severe dietary salt restrictions
could lead to dehydration. If your doctor has you on a salt-
restricted diet, you must have medical clearance to participate in the Two-Day Diet (see Chapter 11).

Diet soda, club soda, mineral water, coffee, tea, and
bouillon are beverages that may be used throughout the
day. If you like to have milk with your tea or coffee, you
can choose low-fat milk from column C of the breakfast
Master Menu and use all or part of it for coffee or tea
throughout the day. There are 8 tablespoons of milk per
each half cup and people usually use 1–2 tablespoons for
each cup of coffee. You may sweeten your coffee or tea
with saccharin or NutraSweet.

On Days: Do's and Don'ts

There are a few general Do's and Don'ts to consider
for On Days. Pay attention to these points to ensure that
you get the maximum benefit from the Two-Day Diet.

- DO drink *at least* three large glasses of water each On
  Day. You will need even more fluids if you are outside
  on a hot day.

- DON'T hesitate to drink more fluids if you feel thirsty or the least bit light-headed.

- DO take a high-quality multivitamin/mineral preparation every day.

- DON'T carry unused food over from one day to another. However, you may save a food and use it in between meals or add it to a later meal on the *same day*. For example, you may save an apple from lunch and have it as a late-night snack.

- DO begin the Two-Day Diet exercise program right away. You may do your On Days exercise at the time of day that is most convenient for you. Remember that your body will lose water when you exercise, so drink extra fluids if you perspire.

- DON'T be concerned if you notice a faint sweet taste in your mouth during On Days. If it occurs, it is a sign that mild ketosis has developed, an expected metabolic effect of On Days. Not everyone will experience a change in taste, but if you do, it will disappear on Off Days and may not return on future On Days.

6.

Off Days

Wednesday, Saturday, and Sunday are all Off Days. During Off Days you will be able to eat more food, eat the kind of foods you naturally crave, and receive a motivational boost that will help you stay on the Two-Day Diet until you reach your weight-loss target. Off Days reverse the metabolic effects of On Days but still promote continuing weight loss.

Men and women follow slightly different plans on Off Days. Men receive approximately 300 calories per day more than women, in consideration of their higher daily caloric requirements. Off Days give women about 1200 calories and men about 1500 calories. Men and women use the same Master Menu for Off Days breakfasts. However, there are separate Lunch/Dinner Master Menus for men and women. A selection of unlimited foods and cravers is also available throughout the day.

OFF DAYS MASTER MENU
For Men and Women

Breakfast (choose one from each column)

A	B	C
½ cup orange or grapefruit juice	2 eggs	¾ cup dry unsweetened cereal
½ grapefruit	1 egg plus 2 strips of bacon	½ cup cooked cereal
1 small orange	1 cup plain low-fat yogurt	1 slice toast
½ cup berries	¾ cup (1% or 2%) cottage cheese	½ English muffin
¼ cantaloupe	1 cup skim or low-fat (1% or 2%) milk	½ bagel
½ banana	1½ oz hard cheese	
	1 heaping tablespoon peanut butter	

OFF DAYS MASTER MENU
For Women

Lunch/Dinner (choose one from each column)

A	B	C	D
1 cup asparagus spears	4 oz chicken	½ cup pasta	1 small apple
1 cup sliced green or wax beans	4 oz turkey	½ cup rice	2 apricots
2 cups bean sprouts	3 oz lean beef, pork, lamb, or veal	1 medium round potato	½ small banana
½ cup sliced beets	4 oz fish or shellfish	⅓ cup lima, vegetarian, or kidney beans	½ cup berries
1 cup chopped broccoli	½ can tuna in water (3¼ oz)	⅓ cup chick-peas	¼ cantaloupe
6 brussels sprouts	1½ oz cheddar cheese	½ cup corn	½ cup cherries
2 cups chopped cabbage	¾ cup (1% or 2%) cottage cheese	¾ cup peas	½ cup grapes
½ cup sliced carrots	1 hard-boiled egg plus 1 oz hard cheese	½ cup lentils	½ grapefruit
		1 slice bread	1 cup diced melon
		1 dinner roll	1 nectarine
			1 small orange
			½ cup diced papaya
			1 medium peach

(continued)

OFF DAYS MASTER MENU
For Women (continued)

Lunch/Dinner (choose one from each column)

A	B	C	D
2 cups chopped cauliflower	1½ cups skim or low-fat (1% or 2%) milk		½ medium pear
1 cup diced eggplant	1 cup plain low-fat yogurt		2 plums
1 cup diced green pepper			⅓ cup diced pineaple
1 cup sliced mushrooms	*or Entree* (plus)		¾ cup tomato or vegetable juice
½ cup chopped onion	2 slices 12″ thin-crust cheese pizza		
1 cup cooked spinach	1 cup chili with beans		
1 cup sliced summer or zucchini squash	1 cup pasta with meat or cheese sauce		
2 medium tomatoes	1 commercial low-calorie frozen entree		
	1 quarter-pound fast-food hamburger		

Unlimited foods such as lettuce, salad greens, and raw spinach may be added as desired. Refer to Unlimited chart.

OFF DAYS MASTER MENU
For Men

Lunch/Dinner (choose one from each column)

A	B	C	D
1 cup asparagus spears	4 oz chicken	1 cup pasta	1 large apple
	4 oz turkey	1 cup rice	4 apricots
1 cup sliced green or wax beans	3 oz lean beef, pork, lamb, or veal	2 medium round potatoes	1 small banana
2 cups bean sprouts	4 oz fish or shellfish	⅔ cup lima, vegetarian, or kidney beans	1 cup berries
½ cup sliced beets	½ can tuna in water (3¼ oz)	⅔ cup chick-peas	½ cantaloupe
			1 cup cherries
1 cup chopped broccoli		1 cup corn	1 cup grapes
	1½ oz cheddar cheese	1½ cup peas	1 grapefruit
6 brussels sprouts	¾ cup (1% or 2%) cottage cheese	1 cup lentils	2 cups diced melon
2 cups chopped cabbage		2 slices bread	2 nectarines
	1 hard-boiled egg plus 1 oz hard cheese	2 dinner rolls	1 large orange
½ cup sliced carrots			1 cup diced papaya
			2 medium peaches

(continued)

OFF DAYS MASTER MENU
For Men (continued)

Lunch/Dinner (choose one from each column)

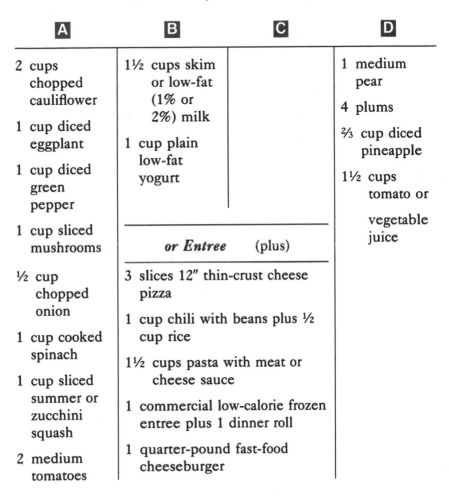

A	B	C	D
2 cups chopped cauliflower	1½ cups skim or low-fat (1% or 2%) milk		1 medium pear
1 cup diced eggplant			4 plums
1 cup diced green pepper	1 cup plain low-fat yogurt		⅔ cup diced pineapple
1 cup sliced mushrooms			1½ cups tomato or vegetable juice
	or Entree (plus)		
½ cup chopped onion	3 slices 12″ thin-crust cheese pizza		
1 cup cooked spinach	1 cup chili with beans plus ½ cup rice		
1 cup sliced summer or zucchini squash	1½ cups pasta with meat or cheese sauce		
	1 commercial low-calorie frozen entree plus 1 dinner roll		
2 medium tomatoes	1 quarter-pound fast-food cheeseburger		

Unlimited foods such as lettuce, salad greens, and raw spinach may be added as desired. Refer to Unlimited chart.

Cravers   *(choose two every Off Day)*

Dairy
1 tablespoon butter/
  margarine
3 tablespoons sour cream
3 tablespoons light cream/
  coffee cream
½ cup ice milk
⅓ cup ice cream/sherbet
⅔ cup milk (regular)
½ cup frozen/fruit yogurt
1 oz cream cheese

Sweets
1½″ square brownie
1/12 8″ angel food cake
½ plain doughnut
½ bran/fruit muffin
2 small cookies
¼ cup raisins
½ small candy bar
4 teaspoons jam/jelly
½ cup fruit Jell-O
6 teaspoons sugar
2 tablespoons honey/syrup

Cocktails
12 fl oz light beer
8 fl oz regular beer
4 fl oz dry wine
1½ fl oz spirits (gin,
  whiskey, vodka, etc.)

Sauces, Condiments, Etc.
1 tablespoon mayonnaise
1 tablespoon vegetable oil
2 tablespoons gravy/sauce
1 tablespoon salad dressing

Snacks
10 potato chips
10 pretzel rings
french fries (½ fast-food
  regular size)
¼ cup plain granola cereal
2 cups buttered popcorn
4 cups plain popcorn
8 small plain crackers

Unlimited Foods *(use as desired during On Days and Off Days)*

lettuce or other salad greens	diet sodas
raw spinach	club soda
radishes	mineral water
cucumber	black coffee
celery	tea, herbal tea
pickles (unsweetened)	saccharin/NutraSweet
horseradish	bouillon, clear broth
garlic	lemon or lime juice
vinegar	salt (in moderation)
diet Jell-O	pepper
mustard	herbs
soy sauce	spices

Breakfasts

The Master Menu for Off Days breakfasts has three columns. A meal is made by choosing one selection from column A, one from column B, and one from column C. Column A foods are fruits and fruit juices. Column B selections are high in protein: eggs, eggs and bacon, low-fat yogurt and milk, cheese, and peanut butter. Eggs should be prepared without butter, margarine, or oil. Column C choices are breads and cereals, high in carbohydrate. Check the nutritional content of dry cereals and pick those without added sugar. Sweetened cereals can be surprisingly high in calories—hidden calories you don't need. You may sprinkle some artificial sweetener on the cereal if you desire.

People who like extra fiber in their diet may want to have high-bran dry or cooked cereals. If you like raw bran, you can combine ¼ cup wheat or oat bran with ½ cup dry cereal instead of having ¾ cup regular dry cereal. See page 145 for a recipe for a delicious oat-bran morning health drink. The Two-Day Diet is naturally rich in fiber through its fruit and vegetable selections, but we certainly encourage the use of bran. High fiber makes good nutritional and medical sense and can prevent the constipation that sometimes occurs when people diet. Regular slices of bread are permitted on Off Days. If you are stocked with very thin bread for On Days, you may substitute two slices of this variety for one regular slice.

Lunches/Dinners

Lunch/Dinner Master Menus for men and women have four columns. A lunch or dinner is put together by choosing one item from each column. In addition, a selection of readily available and popular "entrees" has been built into the Master Menus. These "entrees" combine column B and column C choices. If you would like one of these entrees, simply add one selection from column A and one from column D to complete the meal. Men are permitted more calories than women on Off Days, so many of the lunch/dinner Master Menu portion sizes are larger for men.

Column A selections are vegetables. Unless specified, vegetables can be cooked for hot meals or raw for salads. Column B foods are highest in protein and include main-course portions of poultry, fish, meat, or dairy items. Low-fat dairy products, lean meats, and tuna packed in water are used to minimize calories and fat. Portion sizes of poultry and fish are 4 ounces, and are 3 ounces for beef, pork, lamb, or veal. Remember that these are cooked weights and that these foods lose about 1 ounce of weight in cooking. Refer to Chapter 7 (page 80) for instructions on the preferred method for poultry, meat, and fish preparation. Column C choices are high in carbohydrate. These are foods that are restricted during On Days—pasta, rice, potatoes, beans, peas, corn, lentils, breads, and rolls. All serving sizes of column C foods refer to *cooked* portions. Whole wheat breads and pasta and brown rice can be used to boost the fiber content of your diet.

"Entrees" combine high-protein and high-carbohydrate foods in one dish. The caloric and nutritional content of an entree is similar to a column B plus a column C choice. Our list of entrees has been chosen for your convenience for meals at home or at work. The list includes fast-food items (pizza, hamburgers), common cafeteria selections (chili, pasta with meat or cheese sauce), and grocery freezer selections (commercial low-calorie entrees). Note that quarter-pound fast-food burgers weigh about 3 ounces cooked. There are many excellent brands of low-calorie frozen entrees that contain approximately 300 calories. Most can be popped into the microwave for a meal in a hurry.

Simply add a selection from column A and column D and you have a full Off Day lunch or dinner. Column D choices are fruits, which can be used in fruit salads or as desserts to complete the meal.

Unlimited Foods

The same group of unlimited foods available for On Days is also available for Off Days. Lettuce, salad greens, spinach, cucumber, and celery can be used as the foundation for large salads in combination with Master Menu selections. Two tablespoons of low-calorie salad dressing or lemon juice can be added to each salad. There is also a selection of condiments and beverages for use throughout the day. If you take milk in your coffee or tea, save a milk choice from breakfast and use it throughout the day as we have described on page 64.

Cravers

One recent popular diet book puts the following foods on a strictly "not permitted" list: butter, margarine, syrups, sugar, cream, sour cream, cake, cookies, candy, potato chips, jam, alcohol. These are foods that people love and diet books hate. We call them cravers because most of us have strong natural cravings for foods that are high in carbohydrate and fat. Guess what? The Two-Day Diet permits these kinds of foods, in fact encourages you to eat them in sensible quantities. One of the shortcomings of most diets is their insistence that you radically change your eating habits and forgo foods you especially desire. The chances are, you will not be able to stay on these diets long enough to get close to your weight-loss goal. And let's be realistic.

What is so inherently evil or unhealthy in potato chips or a brownie? Not a thing! The problem lies in the quantity of these foods, not their quality. We believe that a diet that does not permit naturally desirable foods and turns you into a guilt-ridden cheater every time you give in to temptation is a diet doomed to fail. Your cravings for tasty foods are understandable and are not wicked. The trick is learning how to indulge without overindulging. That's one of the lessons the Two-Day Diet teaches.

Our list of cravers includes most of the foods on that other diet's "not permitted" list, as well as many others. The portion sizes are satisfying but not excessive—just enough to kill your cravings without killing your diet. And you are permitted two cravers every Off Day. Have them with your main course, as dessert, or as a between-meal snack. Have two different cravers at different times during the day, or double up and have an extra-large portion of your favorite craver. It's up to you. You can even combine half portions of two cravers to make a whole one. For example, use 2 teaspoons of jam and a ½ tablespoon of butter (one pat) to make one craver to put on a slice of bread.

Some cravers will be used mainly to accompany and enhance the main meal—sour cream on a baked potato, cream in coffee, mayonnaise on a sandwich, gravy on a chop, creamy dressing on a salad, or wine or beer. A number of the Two-Day Diet recipes contain cravers. For example, Eggs Benedict has sour cream and mayonnaise. Braised Fish and Julienne Vegetables is cooked in butter and oil. Other cravers are dessert foods—brownies, ice cream, angel food cake. Still others are classic snack foods—raisins, fruit yogurt, cookies, pretzels, popcorn.

The way you have cravers is entirely your choice. You may use them to have a late-night snack, to have a cocktail or two on Off Days (use diet sodas and tonics as mixers), to create a wonderful dessert like raspberries (from column

D) with vanilla ice cream, or to have some rich sauce with your main course. The most important thing to remember is that cravers are there to be used. *Don't omit them.* They are an integral part of the Two-Day Diet. Off Days are meant to be enjoyable, and cravers help to make them so. If you omit cravers, you may have marginally faster weight loss, but we guarantee that you will be less likely to stay on the diet until you reach your weight-loss goal.

We have been asked whether people are more likely to go crazy and binge on craver foods if they are allowed small regular portions. In our experience, binge eating is most likely to occur when certain foods are totally forbidden on a diet. Temptation and craving build up to a critical threshold until the cravings must be satisfied—one way or another. It's inevitable. And most people will go off a diet completely after one or two binges since the strict regimen is broken and an attitude of defeatism sets in. People simply do not get frustrated on the Two-Day Diet, because their favorite foods are accessible and perfectly legitimate. We do acknowledge that some people have "fatal" weaknesses when it comes to certain foods. Just a bite of a fudge cookie or a nibble on a piece of cherry pie short-circuits all rational thought processes and leads an uncontrollable binge, until the whole bag of cookies or the entire pie is gone. We call this kind of food weakness your Achilles stomach. If you have an Achilles stomach for a particular food, it is best to avoid it entirely. Don't buy it, don't have it in the house. It's that simple.

Off Days: Do's and Don'ts

Here are a few general Do's and Don'ts for Off Days.

- DO take a high-quality multivitamin/mineral preparation every day.

- DON'T be concerned about drinking as much water as you would on On Days. Just drink fluids according to your thirst.

- DO use the Two-Day Diet exercise program every Off Day at whatever time of day is most convenient.

- DON'T save food and carry it over to another day. However, you may save food from one meal and have it later in the same day.

- DO have both your cravers every Off Day, and make sure you eat all the food to which you are entitled.

7.

Making the Most of Master Menus

 The Master Menus achieve a nice balance between simplicity and choice. By choosing one selection from each Master Menu column, you can design literally hundreds of different breakfasts, lunches, and dinners. This chapter will help you use the Master Menus to their greatest potential.

There are two basic strategies for making the most of Master Menus. First of all, use the food preparation techniques that do the most to enhance the taste, appearance, and nutritional value of Master Menu selections. Then combine Master Menu selections into appetizing meals by integrating cravers and Two-Day Diet recipes into menu plans.

FOOD PREPARATION TECHNIQUES

Over the past several years there has been an increasing appreciation of low-calorie styles of cooking. Professional chefs and family cooks alike have realized that a heavy emphasis on butter, oil, egg yolks, cream, and flour in cooking can mask natural flavors and make foods fattening. We strongly advocate the lighter cooking styles and the techniques presented here. They work beautifully with the Two-Day Diet Master Menus.

Vegetables

The best way to prepare fresh vegetables is to steam them. Boiled vegetables lose valuable water-soluble vitamins. If overcooked, vegetables become limp and lose color. Taste, texture, color, and vitamin content are maximized by cooking in steam. Steaming is done with a metal steaming basket, a Chinese bamboo steamer, or in a covered saucepan with a steaming tray. Steaming baskets are inexpensive and well worth the investment.

To steam, clean and cut vegetables and place in a steamer basket. Put one inch of water into a large saucepan and place the steamer basket inside. The basket should stand above the water line, and none of the vegetables should be immersed. Cover the saucepan tightly and bring water to boil over high heat. Then reduce heat and simmer for a few minutes, until vegetables are crisp-tender.

Steaming times vary. For example, spinach leaves cook rapidly, in two to three minutes, while broccoli takes about eight to ten minutes. Frozen vegetables also cook nicely in a steamer. Since they are usually partially cooked before freezing, frozen vegetables require less steaming time.

If you do not have a steamer, you can boil vegetables in a small amount of water—just enough to prevent scorching—in a pot with a tightly fitted lid. Bring water to boil, then reduce heat and simmer until vegetables are crisp-tender. In this way, the vegetables will be partly boiled and partly steamed. Serve vegetables immediately. Do not allow them to stand in water, as flavor and nutrients will be lost.

Another tasty and nutritious way to prepare vegetables for Off Days is stir-frying. Stir-frying is a classic Chinese cooking method that preserves the flavor and texture of food. It is a technique well suited to low-calorie cooking since only a small amount of oil is required for frying. If you are cooking for one, just choose 1 tablespoon of vegetable oil (1 craver) from the cravers list. If you are cooking for two to four people, 2 tablespoons of oil will generally suffice. To stir-fry, use an Oriental wok or a heavy skillet. Heat the wok or skillet over high heat until extremely hot. Add vegetable oil and count to twenty slowly. Then add cut vegetables, tossing and stirring until they are lightly coated in oil. Continue to stir frequently until vegetables are tender and crisp. A small amount of soy or teriyaki sauce may be added during the last few minutes of cooking for a tangy Oriental touch. Serve immediately, piping hot. Off Days portions of chicken, fish, or meat cut into thin strips can be added to vegetables to make a main-course meal.

Don't forget that the way a dish looks is almost as important as the way it tastes. There are several methods for cutting vegetables to enhance their visual presentation. Matchstick-thin slices of vegetables such as carrots, celery, scallions, peppers, and beets are very attractive in salads or in stir-fried dishes.

Poultry

Chicken is a versatile food that is relatively low in calories and cholesterol, hence ideal for dieters. Many of the traditional methods of poultry preparation are low-calorie in approach. Broiling, roasting, and baking require only small amounts of oil for excellent results. Frying is out. Deep-fried or pan-fried chicken is extremely fattening.

Skinning the chicken prior to cooking saves nearly 200 calories per serving, but it does make the chicken dry and less flavorful. To get around this, sear the skinned chicken first in a very hot nonstick skillet brushed with a little vegetable oil. This will seal in the juices and flavor before other ingredients are added. The chicken can be seasoned before it is seared with a sprinkle of salt and pepper or a coating of Louisiana Cajun spices for a fiery-hot taste. When the chicken is browned on both sides, add liquid and other ingredients as desired, reduce heat and simmer. Depending on the dish, chicken stock, wine, canned tomatoes, or other vegetables can be added. The alcohol in wine burns off during cooking, leaving only flavor and aroma behind. Wine used in cooking does not count as a craver. As a rule of thumb, if the wine isn't good enough to drink with enjoyment, it isn't good enough to cook with. Bad wine can spoil a good dish.

Fish

Fish is remarkably low in calories and high in nutritive value. However, you can cancel out many of the advantages by drowning fish in rich, fatty sauces or frying it in batter. Broiling, grilling, poaching, steaming, and baking are preferred techniques for flavorful low-calorie fish cooking.

Fish dishes tend to become dry and tough without the

benefit of butter or rich sauces. The secret of good low-
calorie fish cooking is preventing the fish from drying out.
For broiling and grilling, this can be accomplished by using
pieces of fish about one inch thick. Thinner pieces dry out
too quickly. Pan broil, using a nonstick skillet brushed with
vegetable oil. For oven broiling, lightly oil the oven pan to
prevent sticking. Keep the fish moist during broiling or
grilling with freshly squeezed lemon juice. Broiling and
grilling with lemon juice are also fine ways to cook shellfish.
Always serve fish immediately after cooking.

Poaching is an excellent way to keep fish moist and
tender. Simmer fish fillets, steaks, or whole fish in a covered
skillet. Vegetable stock, fish stock, or water mixed with dry
white wine and seasonings all make wonderful poaching
liquids.

Fish cooks quickly in steam and comes out incredibly
moist and flavorful. Some people shy away from steaming
fish because they think it is difficult to do. It's not, as long
as you have a steaming rack. Simply place the fish on a
steaming rack lightly brushed with oil, put the rack in a
saucepan, heat water to boil, cover tightly, and cook for
five to ten minutes, until fish is flaky and tender.

Baking is the slowest of these cooking methods and thus
the one most likely to need oil, butter or a sauce to keep
fish moist. You can bake fish brushed with a butter craver
on Off Days or smothered in cooked onions and tomatoes
on On Days.

Meat

Meat is naturally high in fat and calories, but it is
certainly possible to make low-calorie meat dishes. Watch
out for inexpensive, fatty hamburger meat. If it's practical
for your budget, use lean ground sirloin. Before you cook

a piece of meat, remove all visible fat with a sharp knife. Oven broiling, grilling, and pan broiling are the fastest and best methods for preparing low-calorie meat dishes. To oven broil, brush the broiling pan with a little vegetable oil to prevent sticking. Steaks and chops should be at least ¾ inch thick. Meat will not usually stick to a grill, so additional oil is not needed for indoor and outdoor grilling. Barbecue sauces tend to be very high in calories and should be avoided. You can add a tangy flavor to grilled meat without adding significant calories by drizzling it with soy or teriyaki sauce. Pan broiling can be done with cuts of meat one inch thick or less. It is unnecessary to add additional oil if you use a nonstick skillet since there is plenty of fat in the meat. Cook the meat slowly, uncovered, over a medium heat, turning occasionally to cook evenly. Pour off fat as it accumulates. If you are using a very lean cut and the meat is dry, add a little beef stock or red wine and cook to desired doneness. Season as needed and serve immediately.

If you choose bacon for an Off Day breakfast, it is best to drain the rashers on paper towels and pat off excess fat.

Eggs

Eggs can be prepared in several ways without adding extra calories. Of course, hard-boiled, soft-boiled, and poached eggs need no butter or oil for cooking. However, eggs can be scrambled or fried perfectly well in a good nonstick skillet without butter or oil. In fact, the natural flavor of an egg comes through brilliantly without the grease. Raw eggs can also be used in blenderized morning drinks. For example, on page 127 you will find a recipe for a banana frappe for On Days breakfasts, with bananas, milk, vanilla extract, and eggs.

Cooking with Herbs and Spices

If you are lucky enough to live near a shop that sells fresh herbs and spices, you can experience the garden-fresh flavors and aromas of fresh ingredients. If you cannot buy fresh herbs and spices, then by all means use dried ones. They also add immeasurable zest to foods and are ideal accompaniments to low-calorie dishes. They complement and augment the natural food flavors and encourage you to savor each bite. Some combinations are perfect marriages of taste: tarragon and chicken, rosemary and lamb, basil and tomatoes. Here are a few tips on herb and spice cooking.

- Cook with one herb or spice at a time until you become familiar with its characteristics. Then experiment with combinations.

- If you buy fresh herbs, you can preserve unused quantities by freezing them in Zip-Lock plastic bags.

- Try to buy whole spices and grind them just before using.

- Store dried herbs and spices in tightly closed containers away from the heat.

- Revive the flavor of dried herbs by briefly soaking them in a little liquid before adding to the recipe.

MENU PLANNING ON THE TWO-DAY DIET

This section describes the kinds of meals you can create using Master Menus, unlimited foods, and cravers. We have created three weeks of Two-Day Diet breakfasts, lunches, and dinners. These sample meal plans include pleasing combinations of Master Menu choices, selected Two-Day Diet recipes from the following chapter, and Off Days cravers.

The sample menus presented here are for *women*. They can be adapted for *men* simply by adding a dinner roll and doubling the fruit portion for each Off Day lunch and dinner. We have not included all the potential unlimited foods you may choose to supplement these menus. That's very much up to individual preference.

Some people find it helpful to do some meal planning a day or more in advance. Appendix II contains menu-planning charts for three weeks of dieting. Each planning chart has a checklist corresponding to On Days and Off Days Master Menu columns. Check the appropriate box for each selection to make sure you have chosen all the foods to which you are entitled. Also list the cravers you want for Off Days. For convenience, cravers are listed with lunches and dinners but you may have your cravers at any time during the day.

TWO-DAY DIET SAMPLE MENUS

Week One: Monday—On Day

Breakfast

½ grapefruit
1 fried egg (fried in greaseless nonstick
   skillet)
½ cup low-fat milk
coffee or tea

Lunch

4–6 ounces baked chicken
½ cup carrots
½ medium pear
beverage from Unlimited list

Dinner

Lamp Chops with Garlic and Rosemary
   (see page 122)
1 broiled tomato
½ cup spinach
½ cup grapes
beverage from Unlimited list

SAMPLE MENU

Tuesday—On Day

Breakfast

Banana Frappe (see page 127)
coffee or tea

Lunch

Open-face turkey sandwich
(1 very thin slice bread, 4 ounces sliced
turkey, lettuce, 1 sliced tomato, onion
slices)
beverage from Unlimited list

Dinner

4–6 ounces broiled halibut
Zucchini and Tomatoes (see page 124)
½ medium pear
beverage from Unlimited list

SAMPLE MENU

Wednesday—Off Day

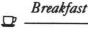 *Breakfast*

½ cup orange juice
½ cup hot oatmeal
1 cup low-fat milk
coffee or tea

Lunch

¾ cup tomato juice
4 ounces grilled swordfish
1 cup sliced green beans
2 small cookies   CRAVER
beverage from Unlimited list

Dinner

---

3 ounces pot roast
1 medium boiled potato
½ cup carrots
Swiss Style Yogurt (see page 141)
   CRAVER (in recipe)
beverage from Unlimited list

SAMPLE MENU

Thursday—On Day

Breakfast

¼ cantaloupe
½ cup 1% or 2% cottage cheese
½ cup low-fat milk
coffee or tea

Lunch

Chef's Salad Deluxe (see page 123)
1 small orange
beverage from Unlimited list

Dinner

1 cheeseburger
  (3-ounce burger, 1 slice American
  cheese)
tossed salad
  (salad greens, 1 sliced medium tomato,
  onion and green pepper slices)
2 tablespoons low-calorie dressing
1 small apple
beverage from Unlimited list

SAMPLE MENU

Friday—On Day

Breakfast

French Toast (see page 127)
coffee or tea

Lunch

2 peach halves
1 cup 1% or 2% cottage cheese
tossed salad
2 tablespoons low-calorie dressing
beverage from Unlimited list

Dinner

Fish Plaki (see page 116)
⅓ cup diced fresh pineapple
beverage from Unlimited list

SAMPLE MENU

Saturday—Off Day

Breakfast

½ cup orange juice
Pancakes and Syrup (see page 145)
  CRAVER (in recipe)
coffee or tea

Lunch

---

4 ounces broiled chicken
1 cup Lentils and Carrots (see page 138)
1 nectarine
beverage from Unlimited list

Dinner

---

2 slices thin-crust cheese pizza
tossed salad
2 tablespoons low-calorie dressing
½ cup strawberries
⅓ cup vanilla ice cream   CRAVER
beverage from Unlimited list

SAMPLE MENU

Sunday—Off Day

Breakfast
_____

½ grapefruit
1 cup low-fat milk
½ toasted English muffin
1 pat butter and 2 teaspoons jam   CRAVER
coffee or tea

Lunch
_____

Crêpes Ratatouille (see page 136)
½ cup diced papaya
beverage from Unlimited list

Dinner
_____

3 ounces pan-broiled sirloin steak
medium baked potato
3 tablespoons sour cream   CRAVER
1 cup asparagus spears
⅓ cup diced pineapple
beverage from Unlimited list

SAMPLE MENU

Week Two: Monday—On Day

Breakfast

½ cup orange juice
1 scrambled egg (cooked in greaseless,
  nonstick skillet)
½ cup low-fat milk
coffee or tea

Lunch

Tuna Fish Salad (see page 118)
1 cup diced melon
beverage from Unlimited list

Dinner

4–6 ounces roast chicken
½ cup spinach
1 cup cauliflower
½ cup berries in season
beverage from Unlimited list

SAMPLE MENU

Tuesday—On Day

Breakfast

1 small orange
½ cup 1% or 2% cottage cheese
½ cup low-fat milk
coffee or tea

 Lunch

open-face combo sandwich
    (1 very thin slice bread, 1 ounce ham, 1
    ounce cheese, 1 sliced hard-boiled egg)
tossed salad
2 tablespoons low-calorie dressing
beverage from Unlimited list

Dinner

Sweet and Sour Chicken (see page 114)
1 peach
beverage from Unlimited list

SAMPLE MENU

Wednesday—Off Day

Breakfast

½ cup grapefruit juice
1 slice whole wheat toast
1 heaping tablespoon peanut butter
coffee or tea

Lunch

1 cup chili with beans
tossed salad
2 tablespoons low-calorie dressing
1 small apple
beverage from Unlimited list

Dinner

1 cup diced melon
½ cup pasta
Tuna Pasta Sauce (see page 134)
one 1½-inch-square brownie   CRAVER
½ cup ice milk   CRAVER
beverage from Unlimited list

SAMPLE MENU

Thursday—On Day

Breakfast
_____

> 1 very thin slice toast
> 1-ounce slice Swiss cheese
> ½ cup low-fat milk
> coffee or tea

Lunch
_____

> ¾ cup vegetable juice
> 4-ounce hamburger
> tossed salad
> 2 tablespoons low-calorie dressing
> beverage from Unlimited list

Dinner
_____

> Tarragon Chicken (see page 112)
> ½ cup carrots
> ½ cup berries in season
> beverage from Unlimited list

SAMPLE MENU

Friday—On Day

Breakfast

½ small banana
½ cup plain low-fat yogurt
1 soft-boiled egg
coffee or tea

Lunch

---

1 cup 1% or 2% cottage cheese
¼ cantaloupe
tossed salad greens
2 tablespoons low-calorie dressing
½ cup sliced beets
beverage from Unlimited list

Dinner

4–6 ounces poached salmon
1 cup asparagus spears
1 small orange
beverage from Unlimited list

SAMPLE MENU

Saturday—Off Day

Breakfast

½ grapefruit
¾ cup unsweetened cereal
1 cup low-fat milk
coffee or tea

Lunch

---

chicken salad sandwich
    (2 very thin slices bread, 4 ounces diced
    cooked chicken mixed with chopped
    celery and 1 tablespoon mayonnaise)
    CRAVER
2 sliced medium tomatoes on lettuce
½ cup grapes
beverage from Unlimited list

Dinner

---

1 cup pasta with grated parmesan cheese
1 cup broccoli
Peach Melba (see page 141)
    CRAVER (in recipe)
beverage from Unlimited list

SAMPLE MENU

Sunday—Off Day

Breakfast

½ cup orange juice
1 poached egg
½ cup low-fat milk
½ toasted English muffin
coffee or tea

Lunch

¾ cup tomato juice
2 meat tacos
tossed salad
2 tablespoons low-calorie dressing
⅓ cup sherbet   CRAVER
beverage from Unlimited list

Dinner

3 ounces roast beef
2 tablespoons gravy   CRAVER
1 medium baked potato
1 cup green beans
1 nectarine
beverage from Unlimited list

SAMPLE MENU

Week Three: Monday—On Day

Breakfast
_____

French Toast (see page 127)
coffee or tea

Lunch
_____

seafood salad
   (4–6 ounces cooked shellfish served on
   tossed salad)
2 tablespoons low-calorie dressing
¼ cantaloupe
beverage from Unlimited list

Dinner
_____

Veal with Mushrooms (see page 121)
1 very thin slice toast
beverage from Unlimited list

SAMPLE MENU

Tuesday—On Day

Breakfast

1 small orange
½ cup 1% or 2% cottage cheese
½ cup low-fat milk
coffee or tea

Lunch

open-face turkey sandwich
(1 very thin slice bread, lettuce, 4
ounces sliced turkey)
½ cup sliced beets
beverage from Unlimited list

Dinner

4–6 ounces broiled swordfish
Oriental Vegetables (see page 125)
⅓ cup diced pineapple
beverage from Unlimited list

SAMPLE MENU

Wednesday—Off Day

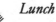

Breakfast

Morning Health Drink (see page 145)
coffee or tea

Lunch

1 cup pasta with cheese
tossed salad
1 tablespoon creamy salad dressing
    CRAVER
1 small apple
beverage from Unlimited list

Dinner

Braised Fish with Julienne Vegetables
    (see page 132)   CRAVER
½ cup rice
½ cup berries in season
beverage from Unlimited list

SAMPLE MENU

Thursday—On Day

Breakfast

    ½ cup strawberries
    ½ cup 1% or 2% cottage cheese
    ½ cup low-fat milk
    coffee or tea

Lunch

    Chef's Salad Deluxe (see page 123)
    ½ banana
    beverage from Unlimited list

Dinner

    4 ounces grilled sirloin steak
    1 cup green beans
    Melon Salad (see page 126)
    beverage from Unlimited list

SAMPLE MENU

Friday—On Day

Breakfast
_____

1 small orange
½ cup plain low-fat yogurt
1 fried egg (fry in greaseless, nonstick
  pan)
coffee or tea

Lunch
_____

¾ cup tomato juice
4–6 ounces baked chicken
1 cup broccoli
beverage from Unlimited list

Dinner
_____

Scallops With Mushrooms and Tomatoes
  (see page 117)
1 peach
beverage from Unlimited list

SAMPLE MENU

Saturday—Off Day

☕ *Breakfast*

½ cup orange juice
½ toasted bagel
1 ounce cream cheese   CRAVER
1 cup low-fat milk
coffee or tea

🍴 *Lunch*

2 slices of a 12″ thin-crust pizza
tossed salad
2 tablespoons low-calorie dressing
1 small apple
beverage from Unlimited list

✕ *Dinner*

Coq au Vin (see page 129)
½ cup brown rice
½ cup grapes
beverage from Unlimited list
4 cups unbuttered popcorn   CRAVER

SAMPLE MENU

Sunday—Off Day

Breakfast

½ grapefruit
¾ cup dry unsweetened cereal
1 cup low-fat milk
¼ cup raisins   CRAVER
coffee or tea

Lunch

Garden Pasta Salad (see page 139)
4 ounces cooked shrimp
1 tablespoon creamy salad
        dressing   CRAVER
1 cup diced melon
beverage from Unlimited list

Dinner

4 ounces roast turkey
⅓ cup lima beans
½ cup carrots
½ cup berries in season
beverage from Unlimited list

8.

Two-Day Diet Recipes

Master Menus give you considerable flexibility and choice in food selection. If you want even more variety in your meals, the recipes that follow can be used to supplement Master Menu choices. Two-Day Diet recipes were designed to offer the same nutritional balance as Master Menu selections. Since On Days and Off Days differ in total caloric content and relative proportion of protein, carbohydrate, and fat, there is one set of recipes for On Days and another for Off Days. You may want to use one of these recipes for a special lunch or a weekend dinner, or you may choose to use these recipes routinely during the Two-Day Diet.

Flavor, color, and texture are all very important in making food attractive. Small portions of high-quality food prepared with creative flair can be as satisfying as large portions of ordinary food. Dishes like Chicken Tarragon and Pork Chops in Creole Sauce can make you forget that you are dieting.

Most of these recipes serve two or four people. Non-dieting family members can supplement their meals, if they wish, with extra portions of the main dish or with side dishes. If you are cooking for one, reduce the ingredients proportionally, or make the full recipe and store the remainder for another meal. Recipes can be expanded for dinner parties and informal entertaining. Dieting should not force your normal activities to grind to a halt, nor should you have to go off in a corner with a special diet plate.

Use the freshest possible ingredients and the best cuts of meat and fish you can afford. The better your food tastes, the less likely you will feel deprived by smaller than usual portion sizes. Large amounts of butter, margarine, oil, or sugar are not necessary to make wonderful-tasting dishes. Instead, recipes have been developed that use steaming, stir-frying, and broiling and that make liberal use of herbs and spices. Low-calorie cooking can become a matter of routine in your life—off the diet as well as on.

How to Use the Recipes

There are recipes for On Days and Off Days. Each recipe is linked to the food columns of the Master Menus. Here is how it works. Sweet and Sour Chicken is an On Day recipe. One portion of this dish provides foods equivalent to columns A and B and that is indicated at the top of the recipe:

A B

To make a complete meal for an On Day lunch or dinner, just turn to your On Day Master Menu and choose one selection from column C—possibilities include a fruit, a glass of milk, or a slice of bread.

Braised Fish with Julienne Vegetables is an Off Day recipe, as indicated at the top of the recipe. One portion of this delicious dish will give you the equivalent to foods from columns A and B, plus one craver:

A B cr

To complete the meal, refer to your Off Days Lunch/Dinner Master Menu and choose a side dish from column C and a fruit from column D. Since only one craver has been used in the recipe, a second craver is available for the day. As always, unlimited foods are available whenever you like.

French Toast is an On Days breakfast recipe. One serving provides the equivalent to foods from columns A, B, and C of the Master Menu for On Days breakfasts:

A B C

This one dish made with bread, eggs, and milk satisfies all your needs for an On Day breakfast!

ON DAYS RECIPES

CHICKEN TERIYAKI   B

2½–3 pounds chicken pieces, skinned
2 cloves garlic, crushed
1 teaspoon fresh ginger root, minced

½ cup soy sauce
1 tablespoon finely grated orange peel
¼ cup rice vinegar

1. Preheat oven to 325°.

2. Place chicken in a baking dish. Mix remaining ingredients together, pour over chicken, and marinate for 1 hour in refrigerator.

3. Bake uncovered for 1 hour or until chicken is tender. Baste several times with marinade while cooking.

Serves 4

TARRAGON CHICKEN   B

2½–3 pounds chicken pieces, skinned
dash of salt and pepper
1 teaspoon olive oil
2 tablespoons finely chopped shallots
1 clove garlic, finely chopped
1 cup chicken stock
½ cup dry white wine
2 tablespoons fresh tarragon, finely chopped
1 tablespoon fresh parsley, finely chopped

1. Sprinkle the chicken with salt and pepper.

2. Brush nonstick skillet with oil. Heat skillet and add the chicken pieces, shallots, and garlic. Lightly brown the chicken for about 10 minutes, stirring frequently.

3. Add the stock, white wine, tarragon, and parsley. Cover and simmer over low heat for 25 minutes.

Serves 4

CHICKEN PROVENÇAL   [A] [B]

12 ounces boneless chicken breasts
1 teaspoon olive oil
dash of salt and pepper
1 clove garlic, crushed
1 stalk celery, chopped
½ cup chicken stock
4 tomatoes, peeled, seeded, and chopped
2 tablespoons fresh chopped parsley
1 teaspoon dried basil

1. Pound chicken breasts with meat mallet until thin. Cut into small serving pieces and sprinkle with salt and pepper.

2. Brush nonstick skillet with olive oil. Heat skillet until hot, then lightly brown the chicken on both sides. Add garlic and celery with about 3 tablespoons of the chicken stock and cook for 2–3 minutes.

3. Add remaining ingredients and simmer gently uncovered until chicken is tender, about 8–10 minutes.

Serves 2

LEMON CHICKEN   [B]

2½–3 pounds chicken pieces, skinned
1 teaspoon olive oil
dash of salt and pepper
½ teaspoon dried thyme
juice of 2 lemons
1 cup chicken stock

1. Preheat oven to 350°.

2. Sprinkle chicken with salt, pepper, and thyme.

3. Heat oil in nonstick skillet and quickly brown chicken on all sides.

4. Arrange in a large casserole and add the lemon juice and stock. Bake covered for 1 hour.

Serves 4

SWEET AND SOUR CHICKEN   🅰 🅱

1 tablespoon vegetable oil
1 pound boneless chicken breasts, cut into thin
   strips
1 clove garlic, finely chopped
3 stalks celery, sliced
½ sweet red pepper, chopped
1 cup bean sprouts
1 8-ounce can unsweetened pineapple tidbits
2 tablespoons vinegar
1 teaspoon fresh ginger root, minced

1. Heat wok or large skillet over high heat until hot. Add oil and count to twenty.

2. Add chicken strips and stir-fry for 2 minutes. Add garlic, celery, red pepper, and bean sprouts, tossing quickly after each addition.

3. Drain pineapple, reserving juice. Toss pineapple with the chicken and vegetables until well mixed.

4. In a small bowl, mix the pineapple juice, vinegar, ginger, salt, and pepper. Pour mixture down side of pan. Mix all ingredients well and serve immediately.

Serves 4

CHICKEN STOCK   Unlimited

leftover carcass of roasting chicken
1 large carrot, coarsely chopped
1 medium onion, quartered
2 stalks celery
3 sprigs fresh parsley
1 bay leaf
6 peppercorns
6 cups water

1. Place all ingredients in a saucepan. Bring to the boil slowly. Simmer uncovered for 1 hour, periodically skimming the fat and foam from the surface.

2. Strain the stock through a piece of cheesecloth or through a fine-screened strainer.

3. Use within 2–3 days, or freeze in ice cube trays for later use.

WRAPPED BAKED FLOUNDER   B

1 pound flounder fillets
juice of 1 lemon
dash of salt and pepper
1 tablespoon fresh dill, chopped (or ¼ teaspoon dill weed)
4 large cabbage leaves

1. Preheat oven to 425°.

2   Sprinkle lemon juice, salt, pepper, and dill over fillets. Set aside.

3. Bring a pot of water to a boil. Drop in the cabbage leaves. Return to the boil and blanch leaves for 5 minutes. Remove

leaves with slotted spoon and pat dry with paper towels. Remove thick part of spine at base of each cabbage leaf.

4. Wrap each fish fillet in one cabbage leaf. Loosely wrap each roll in aluminum foil.

5. Place foil rolls in baking dish. Bake for 20 minutes. Remove foil carefully and serve.

Serves 4

FISH PLAKI   A B

1½ pounds fish fillets (cod, halibut, or haddock)
juice of 1 lemon
dash of salt and pepper
1 teaspoon olive oil
1 medium onion, finely chopped
2 cloves garlic, crushed
1 green pepper, diced
4 tomatoes, chopped
1 teaspoon oregano
2 tablespoons fresh parsley, chopped

1. Preheat oven to 325°.

2. Cut fish into large slices. Place in baking dish and sprinkle with lemon juice, salt, and pepper.

3. Brush a nonstick skillet with olive oil. Heat skillet and cook onions, garlic, and green pepper until softened. Add tomatoes and herbs. Simmer sauce for 10 minutes.

4. Pour sauce over fish. Bake in an oven for about 25–30 minutes, until fish flakes when tested with a fork.

Serves 4

HAWAIIAN SHRIMP KEBABS B C

32 large raw shrimp (about 1 pound), shelled and
   deveined
1 16-ounce can pineapple chunks, unsweetened
2 tablespoons soy sauce
1 tablespoon rice vinegar
1 tablespoon fresh ginger, minced
1 clove garlic, crushed

1. Place shrimp in shallow dish. Drain and reserve juice
from pineapple. Measure one third of a cup of the juice
and mix with soy sauce, vinegar, ginger, and garlic. Pour
over the shrimp and marinate in refrigerator 1 hour.

2. Thread 4 shrimp and 4 pineapple chunks alternately
onto each of 8 skewers.

3. Place on rack of broiling pan, about 4 inches from the
source of heat. Broil for 5 minutes and turn kebabs. Brush
with leftover marinade and broil for an additional 4 minutes
or until shrimp are tender.

Serves 4

SCALLOPS WITH MUSHROOMS
AND TOMATOES A B

1 teaspoon olive oil
3 scallions, thinly sliced
4 ounces mushrooms, sliced
½ cup dry white wine
1 tablespoon parsley, finely chopped
1 pound bay scallops
12 cherry tomatoes
dash of salt and pepper

1. Brush large nonstick skillet with oil. Heat skillet and cook scallions until they soften. Add mushrooms, wine, and parsley. Bring to the boil, then reduce heat and simmer, covered, until mushrooms are tender.

2. Add scallops and tomatoes to skillet and sprinkle with salt and pepper. Cook at high heat, covered, for about 5 minutes or until scallops turn opaque.

Serves 4

TUNA FISH SALAD   A B

1 can (6½ ounces) tuna in water
1 medium tomato, diced
⅓ cucumber, peeled and diced
2 scallions, finely sliced
1 tablespoon plain low-fat yogurt
1–2 tablespoons lemon juice
dash of salt and pepper
a few bibb or red leaf lettuce leaves

1. Drain the tuna fish.

2. In a bowl, mix tuna, tomato, cucumber, scallions, and yogurt. Add lemon juice to taste, and season with salt and pepper.

3. Arrange lettuce leaves on plate and place tuna salad on top.

Serves 1

STUFFED GREEN PEPPERS   🅐 🅑

4 large green peppers
1 teaspoon vegetable oil
1 medium onion, finely chopped
1 pound extra-lean ground beef
¼ teaspoon nutmeg, grated
2 tablespoons fresh parsley, chopped
2 tablespoons chives
salt and pepper to taste
2 cups chicken stock
1 small can pimientos, in strips

1. Preheat oven to 375°.

2. Remove tops of peppers and carefully scoop out seeds and pith. Place peppers in boiling water for 5 minutes. Drain well and gently dry with paper towels.

3. Brush nonstick skillet with oil. Heat skillet and cook onion until softened. Add meat and cook, stirring frequently, until meat has turned color. Drain off fat, then add nutmeg, parsley, chives, salt, and pepper.

4. Stuff peppers carefully with the meat mixture. Place in a casserole small enough to hold peppers upright. Pour chicken stock on and around peppers. Bake for 35 minutes.

5. Drain pimientos. Arrange pimiento strips over peppers in a crisscross fashion.

Serves 4

HAMBURGERS WITH MUSHROOMS
AND PEPPERS   A B

1¼ pounds lean ground sirloin
dash of salt and pepper
4 ounces mushrooms, sliced
1 medium onion, chopped
1 green pepper, cut into strips
¾ cup beef broth

1. Shape meat into four patties. Sprinkle with salt and pepper.

2. Heat skillet until very hot. Place burgers in the skillet and grill 4–5 minutes (or more or less, according to preference).

3. Transfer burgers to a warm platter and cover. Put mushrooms, onions, and peppers into the pan with meat juices and broth. Simmer, covered, until tender.

4. Arrange vegetables around burgers.

Serves 4

OTHER HAMBURGER IDEAS *(use 5 ounces of meat per patty)*

Chiliburgers   B

Add chili powder and cumin to ground meat.

Hamburgers au Poivre   B

Press burgers into crushed black and white peppercorns before cooking.

Cheeseburgers | B

Use smaller burger (4 ounces meat) with 1-ounce slice of cheddar cheese.

Country Burgers | B

Add finely chopped onion and fresh chopped parsley to ground meat.

VEAL WITH MUSHROOMS | A | B

1 tablespoon olive oil
4 veal cutlets (4 to 5 ounces each)
dash of salt and pepper
1 medium onion, chopped
8 ounces of mushrooms, sliced
½ cup chicken stock
1 tablespoon red wine vinegar
1 tablespoon mustard

1. Heat oil in nonstick skillet.

2. Sprinkle veal with salt and pepper. Sauté over high heat for about 3 minutes on each side. Place veal on serving dish and keep warm.

3. Add onions, mushrooms, chicken stock, vinegar, and mustard to the skillet. Simmer, uncovered, at low heat until vegetables are tender.

4. Spoon the sauce over the veal steaks and serve immediately.

Serves 4

PORK CHOPS IN CREOLE SAUCE   🅰 🅱

4 large loin chops (about 8 ounces each)
1 teaspoon vegetable oil
2 stalks celery, finely chopped
1 green pepper, finely chopped
1 medium onion, finely chopped
1 clove garlic, chopped
1 bay leaf
1 16-ounce can tomatoes
Tabasco sauce

1. Trim as much fat as you can from the pork chops.

2. Brush nonstick skillet with oil. Heat skillet and brown pork chops 2 minutes on each side. Add celery, green pepper, onion, garlic, and bay leaf. Sauté vegetables until softened. Add tomatoes.

3. Cover and cook at low heat for 45 minutes or until chops are fork tender.

4. Add Tabasco, a few drops at a time, tasting for desired heat, then serve.

Serves 4

LAMB CHOPS WITH GARLIC AND ROSEMARY   🅱

4 large rib lamb chops (about 8 ounces each)
dash of salt and pepper
1 teaspoon olive oil
2 garlic cloves, chopped
1 cup chicken stock

2 teaspoons dried rosemary leaves
2 tablespoons fresh parsley leaves, chopped

1. Trim all the fat from the chops, leaving only the bone and round of meat. Sprinkle with salt and freshly ground black pepper.

2. Heat oil in nonstick skillet and lightly brown chops on each side. Add garlic and cook slowly, without browning. Add chicken stock and rosemary. Cover and simmer for 15 minutes.

3. Increase the heat and cook uncovered, reducing the liquid, for about 10 minutes. The meat should be slightly pink inside.

4. Add the chopped parsley to the sauce before serving.

Serves 4

CHEF'S SALAD DELUXE   A   B

1 head of bibb lettuce, washed and dried
a few whole leaves of romaine or red-leaf lettuce
2 carrots, grated
2 tomatoes, cut in small wedges
½ green pepper, thinly sliced
½ cucumber, peeled and sliced
2 hard-boiled eggs, cut into quarters
2 ounces sliced Swiss cheese
2 ounces sliced turkey or ham
4 scallions, finely sliced

1. Line a salad bowl with red-leaf or romaine lettuce leaves. Break bibb lettuce into bite-size pieces and layer into lettuce-lined bowl. Add the carrots, tomatoes, green

pepper, and cucumbers and gently toss with the bibb lettuce.

2. Arrange egg wedges around edge of salad.

3. Cut cheese and turkey or ham into thin strips. Arrange strips on top of salad in lattice design.

4. Garnish salad with scallions. Add "vinegarette" dressing or lemon juice.

Serves 2

"VINEGARETTE" DRESSING   `Unlimited`

1 tablespoon dijon-style mustard
½ cup red wine vinegar
1 clove garlic, crushed
1 tablespoon parsley, finely chopped

1. Place all ingredients in covered jar and shake well.

2. Dip a lettuce leaf into dressing. Taste and add a little water to the dressing if the vinegar taste is too strong.

ZUCCHINI AND TOMATOES   `A`

1 pound zucchini, sliced
1 clove garlic, finely chopped
1 small onion, chopped
4 tomatoes, peeled, seeded, and chopped
1 teaspoon dried basil leaves
2 tablespoons fresh parsley, chopped
dash of salt and pepper

1. Place zucchini with onion and garlic in steamer for about 5 minutes or until zucchini is soft.

2. Place tomatoes, basil, and parsley in saucepan and add zucchini mixture. Simmer on low heat for 5 minutes, season and serve.

Serves 4

ORIENTAL VEGETABLES　A

2 tablespoons soy sauce
1 small clove garlic, crushed
1 teaspoon fresh ginger root, minced or ½ teaspoon ground ginger
2 tablespoons fresh parsley, chopped
4 long carrots, sliced diagonally
2 stalks celery, sliced thinly
8 ounces bean sprouts
4 scallions, sliced

1. Mix the soy sauce, garlic, ginger, and parsley. Toss this mixture with the prepared vegetables until they are well coated.

2. Place the vegetables in a steamer for about 4–5 minutes.

Serves 4

GAZPACHO　A

6 very ripe tomatoes, peeled, seeded, and chopped
½ green pepper, chopped
½ small red onion

2 stalks celery
1 cucumber, peeled
1 clove garlic, chopped
1 tablespoon fresh parsley, chopped
1 tablespoon red wine vinegar
salt and pepper to taste
tabasco, if desired

1. Place all the ingredients in a blender or food processor. Process until smooth. Taste and correct seasoning.

2. Chill for a few hours before serving.

Serves 4

MELON SALAD   C

2 cups watermelon scoops
1 cup honeydew melon scoops
1 cup cantaloupe melon scoops
2 tablespoons lemon juice
½ teaspoon fresh ginger, minced or ¼ teaspoon
   powdered ginger

1. Put melon pieces in glass serving bowl.

2. Mix lemon juice and ginger in a cup. Drizzle mixture over melon and toss well.

Serves 4

BREAKFAST DISHES

FRENCH TOAST   A B C

1 teaspoon vegetable oil
1 very thin slice bread
1 egg
¼ cup low-fat (1% or 2%) milk

1. Brush nonstick skillet with oil and heat.

2. Mix egg and milk in shallow pie plate. Place bread in mixture and allow to soak up as much liquid as possible.

3. Place soaked bread in skillet. Pour any remaining egg mixture on top. Lightly brown on both sides.

Serves 1

BANANA FRAPPE   A B C

½ small banana
½ cup skim or low-fat (1% or 2%) milk
1 egg
½ teaspoon vanilla extract

1. Place ingredients in blender with 3 ice cubes.

2. Blend for about 10 seconds and pour into glass.

Serves 1

STRAWBERRY YOGURT SHAKE   🅐 🅒

½ cup strawberries, chopped
½ cup plain low-fat yogurt
½ teaspoon vanilla extract

1. Put ingredients in blender with 3 ice cubes.

2. Blend for about 10 seconds and pour into glass.

   Serves 1

OFF DAYS RECIPES

COQ AU VIN   A B

1 teaspoon vegetable oil
2½–3 pounds chicken pieces, skinned
1 clove garlic, chopped
1 large onion, coarsely chopped
2 carrots, peeled and sliced
4 ounces button mushrooms
1 cup red burgundy wine
½ cup chicken stock
1 bay leaf
salt and pepper to taste
2 tablespoons fresh parsley, chopped

1. Preheat oven to 350°.

2. Brush nonstick skillet with oil. Heat skillet and brown chicken on all sides. Remove chicken and set aside.

3. Add garlic and onion to skillet. Sauté until onions are transparent. Add carrots, mushrooms, wine, stock, bay leaf, salt, and pepper. Cook, stirring, until mixture comes to the boil.

4. Reduce heat, cover, and simmer for 30–35 minutes or until chicken is tender. Discard bay leaf and sprinkle with parsley.

Serves 4

CHICKEN PAPRIKA WITH YOGURT [A] [B]

1 teaspoon olive oil
2½–3 pounds chicken pieces, skinned
1 clove garlic, finely chopped
1 medium onion, chopped
1 green pepper, chopped
4 tomatoes, peeled, seeded, and chopped
½ cup chicken stock
1 teaspoon paprika
½ cup plain low-fat yogurt

1. Brush nonstick skillet with oil. Heat skillet and quickly brown chicken on all sides. Remove chicken from skillet.

2. Add garlic, onion, and green pepper to pan. Sauté until vegetables just start to soften. Add the tomatoes and chicken stock, then stir in the paprika.

3. Return chicken to the skillet. Cover and simmer at low heat for 35 minutes or until chicken is tender.

4. Remove chicken from skillet with slotted spoon to a heated serving dish. Add the yogurt to the sauce and stir over a low heat until well blended. Spoon sauce over chicken and serve immediately.

Serves 4

CURRIED CHICKEN WITH RICE [A] [B] [C]

2½–3 pounds chicken pieces, skinned
1 tablespoon vegetable oil
1 large onion, chopped
1 clove garlic, finely chopped
1 tablespoon curry powder

1 16-ounce can tomatoes
1 cup chicken stock
long grain rice, ¼–½ cup per person

1. Heat oil in nonstick skillet. Quickly brown chicken on all sides, then remove from pan.

2. Add garlic and onions to skillet. Sauté until onions are golden. Add curry powder and cook gently, stirring, for 2 minutes.

3. Replace meat, add tomatoes and chicken stock, and simmer gently for about 30 minutes, until chicken is tender.

4. While chicken is simmering, cook rice according to package directions. Use ¼ cup raw rice for each woman and ½ cup for each man. Serve curry on bed of rice. Women get ½ cup cooked rice; men, 1 cup.

Serves 4

WALDORF CHICKEN SALAD ⬛A ⬛B ⬛cr

1½ cups cooked white-meat chicken, cut in chunks
¼ cup celery, sliced
6 walnut halves, roughly chopped
1 unpeeled medium red apple, diced
½ onion, chopped
¼ cup sour cream
1–2 teaspoons tarragon vinegar
dash of salt and pepper
½ head romaine lettuce

1. Place chicken, celery, walnuts, apple, and onion in mixing bowl.

2. Mix the sour cream and vinegar with salt and pepper.

3. Stir sour cream mixture into chicken salad. Correct seasonings.

4. Chill in refrigerator.

5. Serve chicken salad on romaine lettuce leaves.

Serves 2

BRAISED FISH WITH JULIENNE VEGETABLES   Ⓐ Ⓑ cr

2 carrots, peeled
2 celery stalks
1 green pepper
1 zucchini, peeled
2 teaspoons olive oil
1 tablespoon of butter or margarine
8 ounces thick white fish steaks, (e.g., halibut, swordfish)
salt and pepper to taste
½ cup dry white wine

1. Preheat oven to 425°.

2. Cut carrots, celery, pepper, and zucchini into thin matchstick "julienne" strips. Heat oil and butter in skillet. Sauté vegetables at low heat until they just start to turn color about 2–3 minutes.

3. Remove vegetables from skillet with slotted spoon, reserving the oil and butter. Arrange vegetables loosely in small casserole dish, then place fish on top. Sprinkle fish with salt, pepper, and the reserved oil and butter mixture. Pour wine over fish and vegetables. Cover casserole with lid or foil. Bake for 10 minutes or until fish flakes easily when tested with a fork.

Serves 2

BAKED FISH AND ALMONDS   B   cr

1 tablespoon butter
⅓ cup slivered almonds
1 pound white fish fillets (e.g., cod, haddock)
salt and pepper to taste
1 lemon

1. Preheat oven to 400°.

2. Melt butter in small pan, stir in almonds, then remove from heat.

3. Sprinkle fish fillets with salt and pepper and place on a lightly oiled baking dish. Cut the lemon in half, squeeze juice of half the lemon over fish. Cut remaining half in slices and reserve. Arrange butter-almond mixture evenly over fillets. Bake for 8–10 minutes or until fish flakes easily when tested with a fork.

4. Arrange fish and lemon slices on serving dish.

Serves 4

BAKED STUFFED PORK CHOPS   B   D

4 large rib or loin pork chops (about 1 inch thick)
dash of salt and pepper
1 medium apple, peeled, cored, and finely chopped
2 stalks celery, finely chopped
1 small onion, finely chopped
1 teaspoon ground ginger
1 cup apple cider

1. Preheat oven to 350°.

2. Trim fat from chops. Sprinkle with a little salt and pepper.

3. Mix apple, celery, and onion together in small bowl.

4. Place pork chops in baking dish. Spoon apple mixture over each chop. Mix apple cider with ginger and pour into baking dish around chops.

5. Cover baking dish with foil and bake for 45 minutes, or until fork-tender.

Serves 4

TUNA PASTA SAUCE   Ⓐ Ⓑ

1 teaspoon olive oil
1 medium onion, finely chopped
1 clove garlic, finely chopped
1 6½-ounce can tuna in water, drained
6 plum tomatoes, peeled and chopped
dash of salt and pepper
2 tablespoons fresh parsley, chopped
2 ounces mild cheddar cheese, shredded

1. Brush nonstick skillet with oil. Heat skillet and sauté onions and garlic on low heat until onion is transparent.

2. Chop the tuna with a fork and stir it into the garlic and onion mixture. Add the tomatoes and continue to cook on low heat for 15–20 minutes, stirring occasionally. Add salt and pepper to taste.

3. Add the parsley just before removing the sauce from heat. Serve sauce on pasta and sprinkle with cheese.

Serves 4

PASTA PRIMAVERA   A B C

1 bunch broccoli
1 zucchini, sliced
2 carrots, sliced
⅓ cup frozen peas
4 ounces pasta shells, spirals, bows, etc.
1 teaspoon olive oil
1 clove garlic, chopped
½ cup plain low-fat yogurt
½ cup part-skim ricotta cheese
salt and pepper to taste
2 scallions, sliced
⅓ cup grated parmesan cheese

1. Break the top of broccoli into florets and slice the stem thinly. Steam broccoli, zucchini, and carrots together in steamer for about 5 minutes, until vegetables are barely tender. Rinse with cold water and set aside.

2. Steam the peas over the same cooking water for 2 minutes. Rinse with cold water and set aside.

3. Start cooking pasta according to package instructions. Meanwhile, heat a nonstick skillet brushed with olive oil and cook garlic on low heat until golden. Add the steamed vegetables and heat thoroughly. Remove from heat and set aside.

4. Drain the pasta well. Toss pasta with yogurt and ricotta. Add the steamed vegetables, salt and pepper, and toss lightly. Transfer to heated serving dish. Top with scallions and parmesan.

Serves 4

MEN: Add 1 dinner roll to this meal.

EGGPLANT PARMESAN   A B

2 medium eggplants, unpeeled
1 teaspoon olive oil
1 clove garlic, finely chopped
1 small onion, finely chopped
3 tomatoes, peeled, seeded, and chopped
3 basil leaves
dash of salt and pepper
½ cup grated parmesan cheese
4 ounces grated part-skim mozzarella cheese

1. Preheat oven to 350°.

2. Slice eggplant into pieces about ½ inch thick. Cook in steamer for 20 minutes or until soft. Then drain and pat with paper towels to dry.

3. Heat nonstick skillet with oil. Add garlic and onion. Cook on low heat until onion is transparent. Add tomatoes, basil, salt, and pepper. Simmer over low heat for 10 minutes.

4. Arrange half the eggplant on bottom of shallow baking dish. Spread with half the tomato sauce and half the grated parmesan and mozzarella. Repeat, using the remainder of the eggplant, tomato sauce, and cheeses. The top layer should be cheese.

5. Bake for 35 minutes.

Serves 4

CREPES RATATOUILLE   A B C

1 onion, chopped
1 clove garlic, crushed

1 green pepper, cut into strips
4 tomatoes, peeled, seeded, and chopped
1 medium eggplant, unpeeled and diced
2 zucchini, sliced
dash of salt and pepper
juice of one lemon
½ cup dry white wine
1 teaspoon dried oregano
4 crepes (recipe follows)
4 ounces Swiss cheese, grated

1. Layer the vegetables in a large heavy pan. Add salt and pepper, lemon juice, wine and oregano. Simmer, uncovered, over low heat for 20 minutes.

2. Cook over high heat for 5 minutes to reduce any remaining liquid.

3. Spoon an equal amount of the vegetable stew into 4 crepes. Roll each crepe so that the join overlaps on top.

4. Carefully place the crepes in a shallow baking dish. Sprinkle with grated cheese. Heat under broiler to melt cheese.

Serves 4

MEN: Add 1 dinner roll to this meal.

CREPES

2 eggs
1 cup low-fat milk
½ cup flour
dash of salt
1–2 teaspoons of vegetable oil

1. Beat eggs and milk into a bowl. Beat in flour, a little at a time, and then add the salt. Let batter stand at room temperature for 1 hour.

2. Brush a little oil on a crepe pan or medium-sized nonstick skillet. When the pan is hot, add about ¼ cup of batter and then tilt the pan quickly to cover bottom with batter. Cook crepe until golden brown on one side only. Remove from pan and place on damp towel. Cover.

3. Repeat, using the remaining batter.

Makes 6 crepes

LENTILS AND CARROTS   A C

1 teaspoon vegetable oil
1 medium onion, chopped
1 clove garlic, finely chopped
6 carrots, diced
1 cup washed uncooked lentils
5 cups salt-free beef stock
1 tablespoon dried mixed herbs
salt and pepper to taste

1. Brush nonstick skillet with oil. Heat skillet and cook the onions and garlic, stirring frequently until onions are soft.

2. Transfer to large saucepan. Add carrots, lentils, stock, and herbs. Cook on low heat, uncovered, for approximately 1½ hours. Check occasionally and add more stock or water if necessary.

3. Add salt and pepper to taste.

Serves 4

MEN: Add 1 dinner roll to this meal.

STIR-FRIED BROCCOLI AND CAULIFLOWER

A cr

1½ pounds broccoli
1 head cauliflower
1 tablespoon sesame oil
2 tablespoons vegetable oil
1 tablespoon soy sauce
1 teaspoon sesame seeds

1. Break broccoli and cauliflower into tiny florets. Cut large stems diagonally into ½-inch-thick slices.

2. Heat wok or skillet over high heat for 30 seconds, swirl in sesame and vegetable oil, count to 20, then add the broccoli and cauliflower. Stir-fry until broccoli turns very dark green.

3. Stir in the soy sauce and sesame seeds and serve immediately.

Serves 4

GARDEN PASTA SALAD

A C

4 ounces pasta shells, spirals, bows, etc.
1 teaspoon olive oil
1 bunch broccoli
1 pint cherry tomatoes
½ cucumber, peeled and sliced
4–6 scallions, sliced
salt and pepper to taste

1. Cook pasta al dente, according to package instructions, adding oil to boiling water. Drain well and pat off any excess moisture with a paper towel. Put pasta in large bowl.

2. Break broccoli into florets. Discard large stem.

3. Bring a pot of water to a boil. Drop in the broccoli florets. Return to the boil and blanch for 4 minutes. Drain, rinse with cold water, and set aside.

4. Toss the broccoli florets, tomatoes, cucumber, and scallions with the pasta. Season with salt and pepper. Chill salad before serving.

Serves 4

MEN: You may have 1½ servings of this dish.

VINAIGRETTE DRESSING   cr

1 teaspoon Dijon-style mustard
2 tablespoons red wine vinegar
1 small clove garlic, crushed (optional)
6 tablespoons fine olive oil
salt and pepper to taste

Combine ingredients in a jar or covered container. Shake well until blended. Correct seasoning.

Serves 6

AMBROSIA   D cr

2 medium oranges, peeled, seeded, and cut into
   small pieces
1 16-ounce can of pineapple pieces in unsweetened
   juice
2 small bananas, sliced
½ cup shredded coconut

1. Mix fruit in small glass serving bowl.

2. Stir in coconut. Chill before serving.

   Serves 4

PEACH MELBA   D cr

   1 cup frozen raspberries, thawed
   4 peach halves (fresh or canned without sugar)
   1 pint vanilla ice milk

1. Press raspberries through sieve to make a purée. Set aside and keep at room temperature.

2. Just before serving, place one peach half in each of four individual dessert dishes, cut side up. Spoon half a cup of ice milk on each peach, then drizzle with raspberry purée.

   Serves 4

SWISS-STYLE YOGURT   D cr

   1 medium apple, diced
   ¼ cup raisins
   1 cup low-fat plain yogurt
   1 tablespoon slivered almonds
   powdered cinnamon (optional)

Lightly blend all the ingredients using a little powdered cinnamon if desired.

   Serves 2

CINNAMON APPLE CREPES   [D] [cr]

2 sweet apples, peeled and cored
¼ cup raisins
¼ cup apple juice
½ teaspoon cinnamon
4 crepes (see page 137)
1 tablespoon confectioners' sugar

1. Cut apples into quarters and slice thin.

2. Combine the apples, raisins, apple juice, and cinnamon in a small saucepan. Cook, stirring frequently, until apples are soft.

3. Spoon one quarter of the apple mixture on each crepe. Fold crepes in half and dust with confectioners' sugar.

Serves 4

CHEESE CAKE   [cr]

¼ cup graham-cracker crumbs
4 eggs
½ cup sugar
1 cup low-fat yogurt
2 cups 1% or 2% cottage cheese
2 tablespoons lemon juice
2 teaspoons vanilla extract
1 tablespoon confectioners' sugar

1. Preheat oven to 325°.

2. Sprinkle a lightly greased 9-inch pie plate with graham-cracker crumbs. Shake plate so that crumbs cover entire surface.

3. Combine other ingredients in blender or food processor. Blend or process at high speed, until mixture is smooth.

4. Pour cheese mixture into the prepared pie plate.

5. Bake for 1 hour or until cake feels firm in the middle.

6. Cool overnight in refrigerator. Sprinkle top with confectioners' sugar.

Serves 12

BANANA NUT BREAD   C D cr

3 eggs
⅓ cup honey
⅓ cup vegetable oil
3 ripe bananas, mashed
1 cup low-fat yogurt
1 cup unbleached white flour
1 cup whole wheat flour
3 teaspoons baking powder
¾ cup oat or wheat bran
¼ cup wheat germ
1 teaspoon cinnamon
½ cup chopped walnuts

1. Preheat oven to 350°.

2. In large mixing bowl, beat together eggs, honey, oil, and bananas until smooth. Stir in yogurt.

3. Sift together the flour and baking powder. Fold into the batter together with the bran, wheat germ, and cinnamon. Stir in the chopped walnuts.

4. Turn batter into lightly oiled and floured 9-inch loaf pan.

Cook in oven for about 1 hour or until toothpick inserted in center comes out clean.

WOMEN: *1 twelfth of cake*

MEN: *1 eighth of cake*

APPLE TORTE   D   cr

1 teaspoon vegetable oil
1 egg
1 cup low-fat plain yogurt
¾ cup unbleached white flour
1 teaspoon baking powder
⅓ cup sugar
½ teaspoon cinnamon
2 sweet eating apples
1 tablespoon margarine, melted

1. Preheat oven to 425°.

2. Brush oil onto a 9-inch pie plate.

3. Blend the egg, yogurt, flour, baking powder, sugar, and cinnamon. Spread evenly in pie plate.

4. Peel and core apples. Cut into quarters, then into thin slices. Arrange apple slices on top of cake batter. Brush top of apples with melted margarine.

5. Bake for 20–25 minutes.

Serves 6

BREAKFAST DISHES

PANCAKES   B C cr

⅔ cup flour, white or whole wheat
1 teaspoon baking powder
dash of salt
½ cup whole milk
1 egg, slightly beaten
1 teaspoon vegetable oil
¼ cup pancake or maple syrup

1. Thirty minutes before serving, mix flour, baking powder, salt, milk, and egg until flour is just moistened.

2. Heat skillet or griddle brushed with oil. Using large spoon, pour batter onto skillet or griddle. When underside is golden, turn.

3. Serve immediately with warm syrup.

Serves 2

MORNING HEALTH DRINK   A B C

¼ cup oat bran
1 small banana
1 cup low-fat or skim milk

Place ingredients in blender with 3 ice cubes. Blend for 10 seconds. Pour into glass.

Serves 1

EGGS BENEDICT   B C cr

1 egg
½ English muffin
1 teaspoon mayonnaise
2 tablespoons sour cream
½ teaspoon lemon juice
salt and pepper to taste
1 ounce slice of ham
pinch cayenne pepper

1. Heat nonstick skillet and fry egg without oil.

2. Toast muffin.

3. Make a mock hollandaise sauce by mixing mayonnaise, sour cream, lemon, salt, and pepper.

4. Place ham on top of toasted muffin. Top with egg, then spoon sauce on top. Broil for about 1 minute, until sauce just starts to bubble.

5. Sprinkle with cayenne pepper.

Serves 1

9.

The Two-Day Diet Fits Your Life-style

Diets that force you to change your life-style dramatically don't work. Think about it. How long will you stay on a diet that requires you to eat the same foods or a protein preparation meal after meal, day after day? How long can you suffer the inconvenience of rigidly fixed menu plans that make it difficult to prepare family meals or eat out? Not very long—probably not long enough to reach your weight-loss goal. Furthermore, diets that force a major life-style change don't work in the long run. As soon as the diet is over, you are left to your own devices and your old eating habits. You have learned nothing about healthful eating practices, and you will eventually regain every ounce you may have lost. That is precisely why the Two-Day Diet has been designed to fit seamlessly into your natural life-style—a life-style that includes family and work responsibilities and social engagements.

FAMILY LIFE AND
THE TWO-DAY DIET

As you have seen, meals made from the Two-Day Diet Master Menus contain nutritious, wholesome everyday foods. It is easy to adapt them to fit the needs of nondieting family members. It is unnecessary to prepare one meal for the dieter and another for the rest of the family.

During On Days and Off Days, prepare family lunches and dinners based on Master Menu column B selections— poultry, meat, or fish. While the Two-Day Dieter completes the meal with column A and C choices, other family members may supplement their main course with extra vegetables, rice, pasta, beans, etc. Serving sizes for Two-Day Diet recipes are geared to the dieter. If a recipe serves four, you should have one quarter of the dish. Nondieting family members can have larger portions if they wish. During On Days, while the family is having dessert you can enjoy a column C fruit choice or a hot beverage from the Unlimited list. On Off Days, join in and have a dessert craver.

Women often tell us that dieting is incredibly difficult if there are growing, hungry kids in the house. They feel they must keep the pantry well stocked with snack foods and freshly baked cookies and cakes. As we have said before, if you have a particular food weakness—an Achilles stomach, which will lead to uncontrollable eating—keep that food out of the house even if your kids love it too. Children will benefit from having fewer high-calorie nutritionally empty snacks in their diet. When you shop, stock up with healthier snack choices such as peanut butter, crackers, milk, fruit, raisins, and natural juices and serve them to the kids. If you like to bake your own cakes, pies, and cookies, make just enough for the occasion. If there are leftover portions, freeze them for later use. It is harder to impulsively attack a frozen brick of chocolate cake than a nice soft one sitting on a cake plate. When baking, remember that taste tests and licking the icing bowl will interfere with the metabolic effect of On Days and will use up cravers on Off Days.

THE WORKPLACE AND THE TWO-DAY DIET

The workplace can be tough on dieters. In some offices, the coffee and doughnut cart passes by a couple of times a day, co-workers may bring sweets to celebrate a birthday, cafeterias and local restaurants may not be oriented to the requirements of diet plans. Most diets simply do not work for the working person. The Two-Day Diet does.

One of the features of the Two-Day Diet is the natural appetite suppression you will likely experience during On Days. This appetite suppression makes it comparatively easy to avoid the pastries at an early meeting or the impromptu piece of birthday cake in midmorning. On Off Days you can certainly indulge and use one or even two cravers on an office snack. One point is especially important: Don't skip breakfast. If you skip breakfast, you will be at an extra caloric deficit throughout the day. Your job performance can suffer, and you may be vulnerable to overeating later in the day to compensate.

For lunch at work, you can bring your own, you can eat

in the employee cafeteria, or you can go to a local restaurant
or luncheonette. The Two-Day Diet accommodates all
three options. The Master Menus were created with careful
attention to the kinds of foods available in the workplace
environs. People who have tried to keep on a diet plan with
fixed meals are pretty much stymied at work. In contrast,
Master Menus give you the flexibility of dealing with cafeterias and luncheonettes. As long as they are compatible
with Master Menu portion sizes, have a sandwich or a large
salad or a hot entree with vegetables. If you prefer, you
can prepare your lunch at home with fresh food or leftovers
and take it to work.

   If you travel frequently, you know that the airplane is a
flying restaurant with a very limited menu. Airline food can
be adapted easily enough to the Two-Day Diet. Most airline meals are variations of the standard meat/fish/chicken
main course, side dish of vegetable, side dish of potato/
pasta/rice, green salad, and dessert. For On Days have the
salad (without dressing), the main course (with as little
sauce as possible), and the vegetable. Omit the potato/
pasta/rice and dessert. On Off Days, have the entire meal
and decide if you want to use cravers for salad dressing,
sauce, or dessert. Most airplane desserts will equal two
cravers. The simplest way to deal with time-zone changes
is to reset your meal schedule to the local time at your
destination. For example, if you are traveling from the
United States to Europe on an evening flight, have an airline
dinner, skip the airline breakfast, and have breakfast,
lunch, and dinner the next day in Europe. Traveling in the
opposite direction on a midday flight from Europe, take
the airline lunch, skip the prelanding snack, and have your
dinner later that evening in America.

SOCIAL ENGAGEMENTS AND
THE TWO-DAY DIET

The joy of eating out is preserved by the Two-Day Diet. Restaurant dining, private functions, business meals, and parties with friends are all easily accommodated. Undeniably, there is more choice available during Off Days and that is why we have structured the Two-Day Diet to have Off Days when you need them most—on weekends. But you can deal with social events quite well during On Days too.

The main thing to remember at these occasions is to watch out for the finger foods! Tasty tidbits before the main course can quickly add up to big calories. It's best to avoid them altogether and to concentrate on the main meal. It is quite unnecessary to announce to your host or hostess that you are on a diet and to ask for special consideration. If your party is on an On Day, have a large salad and a generous On-Day-size portion of meat, fish, or chicken. Decline sauces and gravies. While your friends are having dessert, have some fruit. If your entree at a sit-down dinner party is served with a rich sauce or includes starchy foods as an integral part of the dish, it may well be difficult to avoid eating it without embarrassment to yourself or the host. So be it. Have a smaller portion. The metabolic effects of On Days may not be compromised. Get back on track with your next meal, and don't worry about it.

On Off Days, most people will want to use both their cravers at a party. Depending on your tastes, this generally means choosing alcoholic drinks, sauces, or desserts. In addition, the availability of starchy column C choices greatly expands food choices—hamburger buns, baked potatoes, baked beans, etc. Sunday brunch with friends is a snap on the Two-Day Diet. In fact, it can be the most enjoyable

meal of the week. Just combine breakfast and lunch allow-
ances plus cravers, if you like, for an extravagant dining
experience.

Restaurant dining can be more than a social event; for
some people it's a business necessity. We know many people who have successfully managed three or four business
lunches and dinners per week during the Two-Day Diet.
They have told us that this was the first diet they had
experienced in which dining out was no problem.

Here are some general suggestions for restaurant dining
on the Two-Day Diet.

- Remember that you are the one in control of the
  meal—not the waiter, not your fellow diners, and not
  the menu. You determine what you will eat and what
  you will drink.

- Don't be hesitant to ask how a dish is prepared or what
  ingredients are included. It's not rude; it's smart.

- Assert yourself. Most restaurants will prepare a dish
  the way you want it—fish broiled with lemon and a
  little oil, steak without the Bernaise sauce.

During On Days, fish, meat, or poultry prepared without
butter, oil, and sauces will often be your main restaurant
selection. Roasted poultry, grilled steak, blackened fish, or
fish broiled in a very small amount of oil are all delicious
and acceptable choices. So are most chef's salads that combine salad greens, vegetables, meats, and cheese. Vegetable purees usually have added butter and cream and
should be avoided. Starchy side dishes like potatoes, rice,
pasta, peas, and corn may come with the meal, but it's no
sin to leave them. Soups, with the exception of clear broths
and consommés, should be avoided. Have sparkling mineral
water instead of wine, fresh fruit cocktail instead of cheese-
cake. You should be able to walk out of a restaurant on On

Days feeling satisfied and quietly triumphant. You can have a good meal and keep your diet moving along effectively.

In general, some restaurants are easier than others for On Day dining. Continental and American-style restaurants, grills, and seafood restaurants work well on On Days. Chinese, Mexican, and Italian restaurants are more difficult since starchy foods are often integral parts of main dishes. If you find yourself in a restaurant where it is not possible to make Master Menu selections, keep to small portions, skip dessert, and go back to the diet at the very next meal.

Off Day meals at restaurants are easy to negotiate since the availability of cravers and carbohydrate-rich foods opens up a host of menu options. Small amounts of creamy sauces are permissible, as are entrees that combine meat, fish, and poultry with starches such as pasta with meat sauce, stews, and casseroles. A cocktail or wine with your meal is fine and the dessert menu can be used, as long as you stay within the daily limits. Most restaurant dessert portions are larger than one or two cravers, so if you opt for dessert, you should share it with a friend. If main-course portions of meat, fish, and poultry are larger than allowed on the Master Menu for Off Days, pass the extra portion to your spouse or a friend, ask to have it wrapped to take home, or leave it behind. Just because you paid for it doesn't mean you have to eat it. It's your stomach and your waistline.

10.

The Two-Day Diet Exercise Program

Many people who need to lose weight have a negative attitude toward exercise. They associate it with pain, breathlessness, and drudgery. And why shouldn't they? After all, that is precisely how they felt the last time they participated. People who have not done regular exercise for quite a long time often mistakenly embark on an exercise program at a level beyond their present capacity. They buy new running gear or a stationary bicycle or a health-club membership and suddenly work their bodies to exhaustion—once or maybe twice. Then the motivation to continue regular exercise evaporates as they contemplate another session of labored breathing and sore muscles.

The Two-Day Diet exercise program avoids the demotivating trauma usually associated with getting back into physical activity. It helps you develop a positive attitude toward exercise. The core of the program is an exciting concept: low-intensity, or light, exercise. Light exercise is easy on your body, easy on your mind, but surprisingly tough on fat. The physical and psychological benefits will come quickly as you slip painlessly into regular exercise.

The Two-Day Diet exercise program has these important features:

1. It does not assume that you are athletically inclined or in possession of a great deal of willpower. It is realistic and suitable for anyone, no matter how overweight.

2. It can be followed easily on both On Days and Off Days.

3. It is geared to an intensity that favors the burning of stored body fat.

4. It helps preserve muscle tissue as you diet.

5. It will help you avoid regaining weight after the diet is over.

6. It does not cause appetite to increase. In fact, most people experience diminished appetite for several hours following light exercise.

PLANNING YOUR EXERCISE PROGRAM

First, you must choose those activities that are suitable for your interests and compatible with your schedule. Activities should be convenient and accessible to home or work. You may love swimming, but if it is difficult to make it to the pool, you should not rely on this form of exercise. Activities should be self-paced. You should be able to start slowly and gradually work up to your target level. Many

people choose to exercise on their own, but group activities
such as aerobics classes are fine. Just pace yourself rather
than try to keep up with the other class members.

The ideal exercises for the Two-Day Diet program involve continuous nonstrenuous activity. Intermittent activities such as tennis and softball and strenuous exercise like
fast running or a difficult aerobics class are not recommended. Intermittent and strenuous exercises preferen-
tially burn carbohydrate stores. We are primarily interested
in burning fat. Furthermore, strenuous activities are simply
not appropriate to the early stages of a new exercise
program.

These are preferred activities for the Two-Day Diet exercise program:

brisk walking
combination of walking and jogging
jogging
cycling outdoors
stationary cycling
light aerobics class
light aerobics videotape at home
rowing machine
swimming

You should pick the most pleasant environment possible
to perform your activities. If you choose an outdoor activity,
find an attractive circuit around your neighborhood or a local
park. If you exercise indoors, listen to music, watch your
favorite TV show, or prop a book on the handlebars of a
stationary bicycle. Keep sessions varied to prevent monotony. Change walking routes, exercise indoors one day, outdoors another. Decide on the most convenient time of day

to exercise. There is no standard rule, though sticking to a regular time tends to increase adherence to a program.

WHAT IS LIGHT EXERCISE?

The intensity of exercise—light, moderate, or heavy—can be determined by checking the effect it has on your heart rate. The preferred activities listed on the previous page can be light, moderate, or heavy depending on the amount of effort applied. Light exercise quickens your heart rate from its normal resting rate but does not raise it dramatically. In normal health, your heart can only beat up to your so-called age-predicted maximum heart rate. You might be able to reach this heart rate with extreme exertion, but you could sustain it for only a brief period of time before you would drop with exhaustion. Light exercise aims to get your heart beating at 60 to 70 percent of your maximum heart rate. At this rate, your breathing will be faster but you will not be out of breath. You should be able to carry on a normal conversation without gasping.

Refer to the chart on page 158 to find your target heart rate for light exercise. If your heart is beating faster than the upper limit of the range, slow down the pace (for example, jog slower or walk) or decrease the intensity (for example, reduce the tension on the stationary bicycle). If your heart rate is too slow, pick up the pace a bit. Check your heart rate a few times during each exercise session.

Target Heart Rates for Light Exercise

Age	Heart Rate	
	beats per minute	beats per 10 seconds
20–30	114–140	19–23
31–40	108–132	18–22
41–50	102–125	17–21
51–60	96–118	16–20
60 and over	90–111	15–19

How to Take Your Pulse

The easiest place to find your pulse is at the side of your neck, right behind your Adam's apple. Gently probe this area with two or three fingers until you feel the throb of the main neck artery. Press lightly (on one side only!) and count the number of beats for ten seconds to determine if you are in your designated heart-rate range.

STARTING YOUR EXERCISE PROGRAM

The Two-Day Diet exercise program should be started as soon as you start the Two-Day Diet. *It is medically advisable for all adults over the age of forty to get clearance from their doctor before starting any new exercise regimen.* Your exercise program will have the following structure:

Activity	Duration
warm-up	5 minutes
light exercise period	at least 30 minutes

cool-down   5 minutes
stretch and tone   5 minutes
  exercises

We suggest you do at least thirty minutes of continuous light exercise every day. At a minimum, exercise at least five times per week. The most reasonable days to abstain are Tuesdays and Fridays (both second On Days), when your energy reserves are potentially lower. Having said this, we should note that some people feel even more energetic during On Days than Off Days. A thirty-minute session of light exercise is long enough to achieve substantial benefits, but a longer duration of light exercise is even better. If you have the time and the inclination, carry on. The longer you go, the more your body will delve into fat stores.

The Warm-up Phase

During the warm-up phase, you should gradually work up to your target heart-rate range. Your goal should be to increase your heart rate steadily, not abruptly, and to progressively warm your muscles and joints. Most light exercises do not require separate, special warm-up activities. Just start your chosen exercise slowly and rhythmically. If you plan to have a brisk walk, start with a slow walk. If you are bicycling in the park, start slowly in a low gear. Most good aerobics classes have a built-in warm-up phase. After five minutes, increase your level of exertion, until you have reached your target heart-rate zone. Light stretching and limbering before exercise is desirable in cold weather or if you intend to go jogging.

The Light Exercise Period

The list of preferred activities for the Two-Day Diet exercise program is not all-inclusive. Remember, any activity that continuously elevates your heart rate into the target zone qualifies as light exercise. If you have not exercised for a long time, even gentle exertion will get you into your target zone fairly rapidly. Start your first few sessions very slowly. In the early days of the program, aim to stay at the lower end of your target zone. Later on, aim for the middle to high end. In only a few days, you will notice that it takes a quicker pace or greater intensity of effort to reach your target zone. This is an important and sure sign that the exercise program is achieving its goals—improved performance of the cardiovascular system and strengthened muscles.

After a week or two, you may feel so well that you are tempted to push yourself much harder during some or all of your light-exercise interval. You may feel that it is too easy to stay in your target zone. Resist the temptation. Heavier exercise burns less fat. You will be able to exert yourself more during the metabolic adjustment period and maintenance period, after you have reached your weight-loss goal. For the initial phase of the Two-Day Diet, it is far better, if you like, to extend your light-exercise period beyond the required thirty minutes than to push yourself to exhaustion.

It is certainly permissible to mix two or more activities in the same light exercise sessions. For example, spend fifteen minutes on a stationary bicycle followed by fifteen minutes working out with a videotape. Make sure that the transition from one activity to another is fairly rapid, since your heart rate should remain in the target zone for the entire exercise period.

The Cool-Down Phase

The cool-down phase is the period where activity is tapered off gradually to the pre-exercise level. It is designed to gently return your body to the resting state and prevent the light-headedness that sometimes accompanies abrupt cessation of exercise. Cool-down activities are simply an extension of light exercise activities. If you have been jogging, move into a fast walk for a couple of minutes, then a slow walk for a couple of minutes. Most aerobics classes and tapes have a built-in cool-down phase. When you have completed the cool-down, it is a good idea to perform the stretch and tone exercises listed below.

STRETCH AND TONE EXERCISES

Stretch and tone exercises have been selected to address typical "problem areas"—muscle groups that may have lost flexibility and muscles that may have become weak and flabby. Dieters often are disappointed that following weight loss, their bodies seem to lack tone. Loose abdominal muscles and flabby upper arms certainly aren't attractive. It is best to work on these problem areas while you are dieting, not after. The goal is to take typically neglected muscle groups and make them supple and firm so you look your best by the time the diet is over. Many well-organized aerobics classes include a full complement of stretching and toning exercises. In the absence of this kind of a program, these seven exercises can be done in five minutes to tone the areas that usually need it the most—the abdomen, lower back, upper arms, thighs, and calves. Perform the exercises in the following order:

abdominal curl-up
elbow-knee crunch
lower back stretch
push-ups
upper back and side stretch
hamstring stretch
calf stretch

Abdominal Curl-up

Benefit: Tones and strengthens the upper abdominal area. Stronger abdominal muscles improve posture and appearance and protect the back from injury.

Starting Position: Lie on your back with the knees bent and feet flat on floor. Cross arms in front of the chest, placing hands near each shoulder.

Action: Keeping your chin close to your chest, curl up, bringing shoulders and upper back to about 30 degrees off the floor. Pause for one second, then lower yourself back to the floor slowly. Keep your chin close to the chest at all times and do not let your head touch the floor between repetitions. The first few times you do this exercise, try ten repetitions and see how it feels. Eventually, aim to do twenty to thirty at a slow to medium speed.

Points: Do not try to curl up all the way. Curling up further may put strain on your lower back and will not further strengthen your abdominal muscles. When you have finished the abdominal curl-ups, go straight into the elbow-knee crunches.

Elbow-Knee Crunch

Benefit: Tones and strengthens upper and lower abdominal muscles.

Starting Position: Lie on your back with knees bent and feet flat on floor. Place hands behind head.

Action: Lift shoulders off the floor as in the curl-up and bring both feet off the floor at the same time. Move your elbows forward and touch the top of the knees. Lower shoulders and feet back to the floor as in the starting position.

Points: Concentrate on keeping the lower back on the floor at all times. Avoid pulling on your neck with your hands as you raise your upper body. Start with about ten elbow-knee crunches and work up to twenty to thirty slow repetitions per session.

Lower Back Stretch

Benefit: Stretches out the muscles of the lower back to prevent or relieve low back pain and improve posture.

Starting Position: Lie on your back on the floor.

Action: Place hands directly behind the right knee and bring it gently toward your chest until you feel a comfortable stretch. Hold this stretch for thirty seconds, then repeat with the left leg. Stretch each leg twice.

Points: If you suffer from back stiffness, it is a good idea to do the lower back stretch after rising in the morning and after a long period of sitting or standing.

Push-ups

Benefit: Tones and strengthens the upper body, particularly the chest and back of arms.

Starting Position: Lie down facing the floor. Place hands with fingers spread apart, parallel to each other at shoulder level, a little more than shoulder width apart. Curl toes to maintain a good grip with the floor. Raise your body so you are in a straight line from head to toe.

Full push-ups are too difficult for many women. Start with a modified version. Assume the same starting position, but keep your knees and lower legs flat on the floor at all times.

Action: Lower your body straight down until you almost touch your chest to the floor, then smoothly push yourself straight up again to the starting position. Keep your head, back, hips, and legs in one line at all times.

Points: Try to do about ten push-ups with perfect form initially. Eventually, work up into twenty to thirty per session. If you want to work particularly on chest muscles, place your hands wider apart. To concentrate on the back of your upper arms, keep your hands shoulder width apart, with elbows tucked in close to the sides of your body.

Upper Back and Side Stretch

Benefit: Stretches upper body muscles. Reduces stiffness and tension in the neck and shoulders. Particularly good for people who sit at a desk all day.

Starting Position: Stand with your feet shoulder width apart and knees slightly bent. Extend arms over your head and grasp hands.

Action: Stretch arms upward, squeeze shoulder blades together, and hold stretch for fifteen seconds. Relax and assume the same starting position. Stretch the body over to the right side as far as is comfortable and hold for fifteen seconds. Return to the starting position and repeat side stretch to the left side, holding for fifteen seconds. Repeat each sequence once.

Hamstring Stretch

Benefit: Improves flexibility of the low back and the backs of legs. Increased flexibility of these areas helps prevent low-back and upper-leg injuries and aids good posture.

Starting Position: Sit on floor with legs together and straight.

Action: Keeping your back straight, bend forward and reach out with your arms. Hold a comfortable stretch for thirty seconds, then relax. Repeat this stretch once.

Points: Flex your knees slightly to prevent ligament strain.

Calf Stretch

Benefit: Stretches out the back of the lower legs. Helps prevent muscle pulls and soreness.

Starting Position: Stand about arm's length from a wall. Step forward with your right leg and backward with your left leg. Toes should point straight ahead.

Action: Lean forward, resting forearms and elbows against the wall. Move your hips forward until you feel a comfortable stretch in the back of your left leg. Concentrate on pressing your left heel "into" the floor. Hold this stretch for thirty seconds. Relax, change the position of your legs, then stretch your right leg for thirty seconds. Stretch each leg one more time.

Points: To prevent knee strains, do not bounce while stretching. Calf stretches are also useful before a long walk or jog, especially in cold weather.

TRACKING YOUR PROGRESS

It is helpful to make a few simple measurements of your physical condition before starting the Two-Day Diet exercise program. These measurements will enable you to track your progress in some key areas.

Of course, you will check your weight before starting the diet. Then weigh yourself once a week. Although weight loss is the most apparent goal of the diet, it is not the only goal. In fact, body-weight measurements taken in isolation can be misleading. The Two-Day Diet is designed to preserve muscle while you diet. Some people will actually gain muscle as they lose fat. Since muscle tissue is denser than fat, people who build new muscle may find that their rate of weight loss decreases even though they continue to burn fat. Progress may appear to be slowing when it actually is not. The best way to avoid this perceptual trap is to keep track of some key body measurements. If you reach a stage where your rate of weight loss seems disappointing but you are still losing inches from your waist, abdomen, hips, and thighs, you have nothing to worry about. Lost inches attest to lost fat stores.

Measure the circumference of chest/bust, waist, abdomen, hips, and thighs with a measuring tape against bare skin. Take the measurements standing upright without tensing your muscles. Chest circumference should be checked after exhaling. Waist measurement is taken just above the navel. The abdomen is measured at a point midway between waist and hips. Measure hip circumference at the widest point around buttocks and measure thigh circumference at the widest point. Make these measurements right before starting the Two-Day Diet, then repeat every two weeks. You can track your progress on the chart below.

Charting Your Progress

Starting date _____   Weight-loss goal _____ pounds

	start	1	2	3	4	5	6
Date							
Measurements							
Weight (*lbs.*)							
Chest/Bust (*in.*)							
Waist							
Abdomen							
Hips							
Thighs							

When You Have Reached Your Weight-Loss Goal

When you reach your target weight-loss goal, you will enter the Two-Day Diet metabolic adjustment period. During this two-week period, the nature of the diet and the nature of the exercise program change. This special period is designed to prevent the weight regain that dieters often experience as they make the transition into a maintenance program. The exercises for the metabolic adjustment and maintenance periods are described in Chapters 12 and 13. They build naturally on progress made during the light-exercise program. Most important, these exercise programs will help you keep the fat off permanently.

11.

Special Considerations for Women and People with Medical Conditions

The decision to go on a diet carries a responsibility with it. That responsibility is to *yourself*. You must be confident you are doing everything possible to ensure your weight loss is safe and healthful. You *can* be confident that the Two-Day Diet is a safe route to accelerated weight loss. We have included this section to provide additional information for people with special nutritional and medical requirements. This information is not a substitute for consultation with your personal physician. *If you have an underlying medical problem for which you are under a doctor's care, check with him or her before starting the Two-Day Diet.*

WOMEN

Women have special nutritional requirements that must be considered when contemplating a diet. Pregnancy and breast-feeding place extraordinary metabolic stresses on the body, and it is important to know when to diet and when not to. Women are also prone to certain nutritional deficiencies. These, however, are avoidable.

Pregnancy and Breast-Feeding

Weight gain during pregnancy is necessary to support the nutritional requirements of the growing fetus. A normal gestation requires a total of energy cost of approximately 75,000 calories. Typically, a woman will gain about twenty-five pounds. Caloric energy is also required to produce the milk needed for breast-feeding. Except in cases of truly excessive weight gain, the period of pregnancy and post-partum breast-feeding is *not* the time to go on *any* diet. If your obstetrician feels you have excessive weight gain, you will be placed on a medically supervised, individualized diet.

Breast-feeding may be regarded as a natural weight-reducing activity. Milk production uses up about 800 calories per day of stored fuel reserves. Most women will gradually lose their extra pounds in the postpartum period as they get back to their normal activity patterns and eating habits. Unfortunately, some women have difficulty returning to their baseline weight, retaining persistent pounds with each pregnancy. The time to consider dieting is a couple of weeks after breast-feeding is finished and the body has had a chance to return to its usual metabolic state. If you think you need to lose weight at this point, the Two-

Day Diet is an excellent way to do so. If you are unsure if you need to diet, ask your obstetrician.

Iron Requirements

Women of childbearing age have a greater need for iron in their diet to compensate for monthly losses of the mineral through menstruation. It is usually recommended that adult women receive 18 milligrams of iron daily to prevent iron-deficiency anemia. Iron-rich foods include liver, pork, beef, dried fruit, leafy vegetables, and enriched breads and cereals. A balanced diet typically supplies only 6 milligrams of iron per 1000 calories. For this reason, many women rely on supplements to fulfill daily needs, especially during a calorie-restricted diet. Although there are many iron-rich foods available on the Two-Day Diet, we recommend that you take daily a high-quality multivitamin/mineral preparation. This will make up for the iron deficit imposed by a low-calorie diet. There is usually no need to take a separate iron supplement.

Calcium Requirements

Dietary calcium is essential for maintaining the development of bones and reducing the risk for osteoporosis, a bone-thinning condition affecting women after their menopause. Osteoporosis is a major public-health problem. Over 20 million American women are afflicted by this disease, which renders the bones brittle and vulnerable to fracture.

Although it usually causes serious problems only after the fifth decade, calcium loss progresses steadily throughout life. To prevent osteoporosis from developing later in life, it is advisable for women especially to pay careful attention to daily calcium intake. Right now, the recommended daily allowance of calcium is 800 milligrams per day, although some experts believe that 1000 to 1500 would be more prudent. There are some practical problems in obtaining 1000 milligrams of calcium from food sources alone. You would have to eat the equivalent of one cup of low-fat milk, one ounce of cheese, one cup of plain yogurt, and one cup of broccoli daily to reach this level. Dairy foods and dark leafy vegetables, the richest dietary sources of calcium, are abundantly available for both On Day and Off Day meals. It is certainly possible to have a diet rich in calcium by consistently making high-calcium Master Menu selections, and we encourage women to do so. However, you will need to take a daily calcium supplement to make sure you consistently reach target calcium levels. Some multivitamin/ mineral preparations have special formulas for women that supply the daily calcium requirement, but you will probably do better taking specific calcium supplements. Ask your pharmacist or doctor to recommend some good products.

DIABETES

There are two types of diabetes. Juvenile-onset diabetes typically develops in the first two decades of life. The pancreas glands of juvenile diabetics fail to produce adequate insulin hormone and they must rely on daily life-sustaining insulin injections. They are usually not overweight and generally do not require weight-reduction diets.

The second type of diabetes usually develops later in life and is often called maturity-onset diabetes. This is by far the most common type. Maturity-onset diabetics are often overweight. Although their pancreas glands produce an adequate amount of insulin, their extra body fat impairs the efficiency of insulin action. Maturity-onset diabetics have inappropriately high blood-sugar levels throughout much of the day, especially after meals. Elevated blood sugar produces a host of troubling acute symptoms such as fatigue, excessive thirst, urination, and hunger and can lead to serious long-term effects on the eyes, heart, kidneys, and blood vessels.

Oral medications can lower blood sugar by making the cells of the body more responsive to the effects of insulin. Some adult-onset diabetics who fail to respond adequately to these medications are given insulin injections, but the basic therapy for any maturity-onset diabetic who is overweight is first to *lose weight*. Many overweight diabetics who successfully trim down can normalize their blood sugar and thereafter do not require medications.

Few medical authorities would dispute that weight reduction is the primary therapy for overweight maturity-onset diabetics and that diet therapy should be tried before medications are prescribed. One thing is certain: *Diet therapy for diabetes must be medically supervised, ideally under the auspices of a registered dietician. The Two-Day Diet and exercise program may be well suited for certain overweight diabetics, but that is for your doctor and dietician to decide.*

HYPERTENSION

Hypertension, or elevated blood pressure, is a leading cause of cardiovascular disease and death, affecting approximately one in every six adults in America. It is a particular problem among black Americans. Not all individuals with hypertension are overweight, but those who are may have improvement or normalization of blood pressure with weight reduction.

With the exception of those individuals with markedly elevated blood pressure, who clearly require drug therapy, most physicians will try diet therapy and salt reduction as the initial steps for mild hypertensives. If these interventions fail to reduce blood pressure to a desirable level, then antihypertensive medications are prescribed. A variety of drugs may be used, including diuretics, agents that eliminate sodium and water from the body.

If you are under a doctor's care for hypertension, your weight loss should be medically supervised. The Two-Day Diet may be ideal for some people with high blood pressure, but we must sound a cautionary note. *If you are on a salt-restricted diet and take a diuretic medication, the extra fluid losses incurred by On Days could cause light-headedness or even fainting. This also applies to individuals on diuretics for other medical conditions. Your doctor must decide if this diet is safe for you.*

ELEVATED CHOLESTEROL

Elevation of blood cholesterol and/or certain blood fats (lipids) is a clear risk factor for the development of heart attack and stroke. If you have these elevations, you should take measures to reduce them. Even if your levels are in the normal range, it is prudent to place some limitations on the amount of fat and cholesterol in your diet.

The primary therapy for elevated cholesterol and lipids is dietary, including some restriction of cholesterol-laden foods. Organ and red meats, eggs, whole milk and cheese, butter, ice cream, and mayonnaise are limited. The use of fish, poultry, vegetables, fruits, cereals, low-fat milk, and low-fat cheeses is encouraged. People with significant elevations in cholesterol are often placed on highly restrictive diets and may have to use cholesterol- and lipid-lowering medications.

Many nutritional authorities, including the American Heart Association, believe it is sensible for most adults to place a 300-milligram-daily limit on cholesterol intake. One egg yolk contains about 275 milligrams of cholesterol! Four ounces of beef, lamb, pork, or veal contain about 100 milligrams each. It is obvious that some limits need to be placed on egg and red meat consumption to keep your cholesterol intake at an acceptable daily level.

Two-Day Diet Master Menus have low-cholesterol choices available for all meals. If you need to restrict cholesterol in your diet, Master Menus give you the flexibility of consistently making low-cholesterol choices, avoiding or restricting eggs, red meat, and cheese. Even if you do not have a problem, keeping your egg consumption to three per week is a good idea.

HEART DISEASE

The Two-Day Diet exercise program is not strenuous. *Nevertheless, individuals with known or suspected heart disease— like those with angina (chest pain due to limitation of blood flow to heart muscle) or those who have suffered a heart attack in the past—should embark on the exercise program only after careful consultation with their primary physician or cardiologist.*

In addition, all adults over the age of forty contemplating this exercise program should have a thorough medical screening exam. Your physician will examine you and run some simple tests. You will be asked whether you get chest discomfort or unusual shortness of breath with exertion, whether you ever get palpitations or dizziness. Inquiries will be made about diseases you may have had in the past, your history of cigarette smoking, and about family members with heart disease. A physical examination will focus on the status of your heart, lungs, and peripheral blood vessels. You will receive an electrocardiogram, perhaps a chest X ray, a battery of standard blood tests, and maybe even an exercise-stress test to see how your heart performs during exercise. After this examination, follow the advice of your physician.

ARTHRITIS

Degenerative arthritis, also known as osteoarthritis, may develop as an unfortunate complication of long-standing severe obesity. A disease of wear and tear, it often affects the joints that bear the brunt of excessive body weight, especially the hips and knees. The normal smooth joint surfaces at the interface of two bones are literally ground down, resulting in swelling, inflammation, and loss of joint mobility. If the arthritis progresses to an advanced state, surgical replacement of the joint may be required. Weight reduction is often critically important in cases of degenerative arthritis. If you have degenerative arthritis and no other condition that would preclude your participation, the Two-Day Diet and exercise program should serve you well. Exercising with degenerative arthritis can be challenging. *Many activities may be too painful and exercises such as jogging, even if tolerable, could further damage eroded joints.* Swimming is perhaps the ideal exercise for people with degenerative arthritis, since it places minimal strain on joints.

INTESTINAL DISORDERS

Certain diseases of the large intestine may be aided by a high-fiber diet. Diverticular disease, a condition where balloon-shaped pouches form in the walls of the large intestine, and irritable colitis, a condition causing cramping and diarrhea, may be improved by increasing the amount of dietary fiber. If your doctor has advised a high-fiber diet, you should be able to get it on the Two-Day Diet. Choose high-bran cereals for breakfast every Off Day. Consistently choose vegetables high in fiber, such as green beans, brussels sprouts, cauliflower, peas, and squash and fruits like apples, pears, and blackberries. Whole wheat bread and crackers have more fiber than those baked with white flour. *If you are not sure that you will receive enough fiber on the diet to keep your condition under control, check with your doctor or dietician.*

12.

The Metabolic Adjustment Period—
Adjusting to Your New Weight

When you have reached your target weight-loss goal, you have reached the most critical stage of your diet. This is the point where dieters are most vulnerable to weight regain. And this is why the Two-Day Diet includes the metabolic adjustment period to allow the dieter to adjust gradually to his or her new weight without regaining shed pounds. A case in point: Michael, a forty-two-year-old journalist, lost almost forty pounds on a medically supervised liquid protein diet. As he was losing this weight he did not feel vigorous enough to exercise, and in fact, exercise was not prominently featured in his particular diet program. When he got very close to his original goal of forty pounds of weight loss, he was switched back to real food and threw a party to celebrate. Although he was given detailed instructions on how to deal with real food he got complacent, stopped going to his clinic appointments, and resumed many of his old eating habits. It took him ten weeks to lose the weight and only seven weeks to gain it all back. He fell victim to the condition obesity researchers call the repletion reaction. Michael's experience is not the exception among dieters. Unfortunately, it is closer to the rule.

THE REPLETION REACTION

One of the dieter's main enemies is a complex chain of metabolic events that favor refilling the fat stores depleted during a diet. Earlier, we mentioned the set-point theory, which proposes that the body tends to maintain its weight at a certain level. Let's say your long-term baseline weight is 150 pounds but you successfully diet to 130 pounds. If you let nature take its course, your body will defend its natural set point of 150 pounds and efficiently "help" you regain the twenty pounds. At least your body "thinks" it is helping you overcome your admittedly self-imposed food deprivation. It does so via the repletion reaction.

Experiments with rats have given obesity researchers an insight into the mechanism of the repletion reaction. When rats are deliberately overfed, their fat cells enlarge and become packed with fat droplets. At some point there is simply no more storage space available. In response to the need for additional storage space, the animal is capable of forming new fat cells. Once formed, they become permanent.

The overfed rat is left with a greater number of fat cells than it had originally. If a fast is imposed, these fat cells can be made to shrink but not to disappear. However, they are able to fill up with fat again and are exceptionally prone to do so. Refeeding animals after a period of caloric restriction leads to a metabolic state whereby the re-formation of fat is greatly facilitated. Fat cells swell and rats quickly plump up.

The implications for human dieters are clear. Over the period of time you have become overweight your fat cells have enlarged and, if the experimental data is correct, multiplied. Dieting can shrink these fat cells, but when the diet ends, the repletion reaction starts. You may experience greater hunger and superefficiently convert food into fat. Like tiny dry sponges doused in water, your fat cells are liable to fill up with fat again, leading to rapid weight regain.

DEFEATING THE REPLETION REACTION

If you carefully follow all aspects of the Two-Day Diet and exercise program, by the time you reach your target weight-loss goal, you will have already gone a long way toward defeating the repletion reaction.

The Two-Day Diet Exercise Program counteracts the natural fall in metabolic rate produced by dieting. It does so via short-term and long-term effects. In the short-term, light exercise can produce a measurable boost in metabolic rate for a period of time, not only during but *after* the exercise has been completed. This postexercise effect will vary from person to person depending on an individual's body chemistry, type, and the duration of activity. However, the effect can last up to a full twenty-four hours after exercise. In the long term, the Two-Day Diet and exercise program decreases body fat and preserves or even builds muscle tissue. To put it simply, you will be a leaner individual by the time you reach your weight-loss goal. Since muscle tissue at rest burns more calories than fat tissue, your resting metabolic rate will increase. You will burn more calories at rest, convert less food to fat, and be in a better position to avoid repleting your fat storage compartment.

As you prepare to make the change from the active dieting phase of the Two-Day Diet to the maintenance phase, you will have several factors working in your favor:

1. You will not be emerging from a starvation diet and a state of chronic hunger. People who come off very low calorie diets often have trouble controlling themselves when calories are increased. The Two-Day Diet provides you with enough food to avoid feelings of hunger and deprivation.

2. You will not have to cope with the transition to normal food from a diet that has been based on special foods and drinks. This kind of transition can be extremely difficult, often resulting in overeating as soon as good-tasting normal food is reintroduced.

3. You will have raised your metabolic rate with the Two-Day Diet and exercise program.

Still, the repletion reaction is a powerful foe. To make sure you are able to conquer it, we have created a special two-week program specifically designed to prevent weight regain and to ease you into the maintenance phase. We call this program the metabolic adjustment period.

THE METABOLIC ADJUSTMENT PERIOD

This period allows your body to adjust to a greater caloric intake. You will not experience the repletion reaction and you will not gain weight. Start this program as soon as you have reached your weight-loss goal. Some people may actually lose an additional few pounds during this period, especially if they have achieved their weight loss quickly and are not habitual dieters.

The time it has taken to reach your weight-loss target will vary considerably among individuals. It is dependent upon age, sex, amount of weight to be lost, length of time you have been overweight, history of previous dieting, and genetic factors. We noted in Chapter 4 that most people will get to their target in two to six weeks. If you need to lose a large amount of weight, thirty pounds or more, you may remain on the Two-Day Diet for as long as it takes to achieve your goal. It is perfectly safe to stay on the program for extended periods of time. However, it is acceptable to lose weight in stages if you prefer, say twenty pounds at a time. *If you choose a staged approach, it is important to enter the metabolic adjustment period after each stage.* Stabilize your new weight, maintain it for a while, then go back on the Two-Day Diet and carry on the weight loss.

The metabolic adjustment period incorporates a two-pronged attack against weight regain. There is a diet component and an exercise component. After two weeks on this program, you will be in an excellent position physically and mentally to enter the long-term phase of weight maintenance.

The Diet Component

Off Day plans form the core of the metabolic adjustment period diet program. Men and women will use their respective Off Days Master Menus for breakfast, lunch, and dinner *every* day of the two week period. *On Days Master Menus are not to be used.*

Week One: During the first week follow Off Day meal plans exactly as described in Chapter 6. This means making full use of Master Menus, Off Day recipes, cravers, and unlimited foods. Women will receive approximately 1200 calories, men approximately 1500 calories per day.

Week Two: During week two you will further increase your daily calories in a healthful, controlled fashion. Continue to follow Off Day meal plans—with one exception. For lunches and dinners, increase the portion sizes of column A vegetable dishes and column D fruit choices. How much is too much? There are no hard and fixed rules. Column A and D selections are fairly low in calories and high in nutritional value. You can increase these fruits and vegetables considerably —certainly, to double or triple the original size. Let your appetite be your guide. Column B and C portion sizes remain unchanged. So do cravers; keep to two of them per day.

There are three important guidelines to ensure that the diet program for the metabolic adjustment period successfully prepares you for the maintenance period:

1. Watch out for salty foods, and avoid the salt shaker. When you have been on a diet and then start increasing calories, there is a natural and often strong tendency for the body to retain salt and water. This can lead to bloating and water weight, especially in women. You need to carefully avoid salty foods during the metabolic adjustment period. Limit processed meats, cheeses, soy sauce and other condiments, pretzels, potato chips, and bouillon. Also, add very little salt to your food in cooking.

2. Cravers are now allowed every day, but avoid or limit
   sugary cravers. Foods that are high in sugar seem to
   augment the repletion reaction and increase hunger. Use
   cravers like vegetable oils for cooking and salads, un-
   salted crackers, popcorn, and dairy cravers such as sour
   cream and whole milk.

3. Weigh yourself every three to four days. If your weight
   is creeping up and you feel you are retaining water (abdominal bloating, tight rings, tight shoes), further reduce
   your salt consumption. If the weight gain does not seem
   to be caused by water retention, cut back on the cravers
   and consider whether you have been careful with portion
   sizes and faithful to your exercise program.

The Exercise Component

The exercise program for the metabolic adjustment
period also helps combat the repletion reaction and prepares
you for the maintenance period ahead. During light exercise, you have aimed for a heart rate of 60 to 70 percent of
your age-predicted maximum heart rate. You will now aim
for a heart rate in the range of 70 to 85 percent of maximum.
This level of intensity is called moderate exercise.

Graduating to a higher intensity of exercise during the
metabolic adjustment period means that you will have a
greater postexercise boost in your metabolic rate and you
will increase muscle tissue in exercising areas. Your body
composition will continue to shift toward increasing lean-
ness, further increasing your metabolic rate.

You should engage in moderate exercise at least five times
a week during the metabolic adjustment period. Choosing
activities for moderate exercise is easy: the same activities

you have used for light exercise qualify. The only difference is that you will exert yourself a little more. If you have been doing light exercise with a combination of walking and jogging, you may now need mostly to jog. If you have been cycling, you will need to increase the tension or workload. If you have been taking it easy in an aerobics class, you will need to work harder or increase your pace. These are your new heart-rate goals:

Target Heart Rates for Moderate Exercise

Age	Heart Rate	
	beats per minute	beats per 10 seconds
20–30	133–170	22–28
31–40	126–161	21–27
41–50	119–152	20–25
51–60	112–144	19–24
61 and over	105–135	18–23

Initially, try to keep your heart rate in the lower end of your new target zone. This should be fairly easy for you since the upper end of your target zone for light exercise overlaps with the lower end for moderate exercise.

The program for the metabolic adjustment period has a smiliar structure as your previous exercise program:

Activity	Duration
warm-up	5 minutes
moderate exercise period	at least 30 minutes

cool-down   5 minutes
stretch and tone   5 minutes
  exercises

Follow the same principles of warming up and cooling down before and after exercising that we described in Chapter 10. Also, continue to do the seven stretch and tone exercises. Most people become particularly aware of weak and flabby muscles after they have lost weight, so you should continue to work on flexibility and toning.

13.

The Maintenance Period—
Maintaining Your New Weight

By the time you have arrived at the Two-Day Diet maintenance period:

- You will have reached your target weight-loss goal.
- You will be a leaner person with a lower proportion of body fat.
- You will have significantly improved your fitness level and cardiovascular health.
- You will look better and feel terrific.

and

- You will have learned the "secrets" of long-term weight maintenance.

This last point may surprise you. After all, we haven't yet discussed the subject of weight maintenance. Nevertheless, *people who follow the Two-Day Diet will be learning the techniques of long-term weight control as they go along.*

Why is long-term weight control so important? Repeating cycles of weight loss and weight regain—the yo-yo or roller-coaster effect—are harmful. The sad fact is that when people lose weight and put it back on, they usually wind up with more fat than when they started. Unlike the Two-Day Diet, most diets cause both fat and muscle to be lost. When the diet ends, almost all the weight regained is fat. Also, with each successive attempt to diet, losing weight gets harder and weight loss is slower. And to top it off, recent research indicates that people who start with fat around the lower body, hips and thighs, tend to regain it around the abdomen. Abdominal fat seems to carry a greater risk of heart disease than lower body fat, so this is another potentially worrisome situation. The message is clear: Once you take weight off, keep it off.

The "secrets" of long-term weight maintenance aren't really secrets at all. They are actually easily understood principles based on state-of-the art research in nutritional science and physical fitness. As you will see, these principles follow logically from earlier phases of the Two-Day Diet and exercise program.

DIET AND WEIGHT MAINTENANCE

In the initial weight-loss phase, the Two-Day Diet is deliberately unbalanced during On Days to exploit the rapid fat-burning metabolic aspects of a low-carbohydrate high-protein regimen. Once the desired amount of weight has been lost, the diet becomes more balanced. The metabolic adjustment period exclusively uses Off Days. Off Days have a more balanced proportion of protein, carbohydrate, and fat. The metabolic effects of On Days are no longer required at this point. During the second week of the metabolic adjustment period, the diet becomes even more balanced as portion sizes of vegetables and fruits are increased. The maintenance period takes the final step and fully balances the diet according to the most recent recommendations of nutritional authorities.

You should regard Off Day meal plans as the foundation for your maintenance program. Off Day breakfasts require no modifications to be ideal meals for a maintenance plan. If you check the Off Days Master Menu, you will see that breakfasts are varied, ample and sustaining, without excessive calories. Remember the importance of controlling your weekly consumption of eggs. Given that caveat, Off Day breakfasts will serve you well in your effort to preserve your weight loss.

With simple modifications, Off Day lunches and dinners become excellent meals for long-term maintenance. During the metabolic adjustment period, portion sizes of Master Menu column A vegetables and column D fruits are increased according to preference and appetite. For weight maintenance, we encourage you to continue eating generous portions of vegetables and fruits with lunch and dinner and to choose fresh fruit for snacks.

Portion sizes of column C carbohydrate-rich dishes also should increase during the maintenance period. Rice, pasta, beans, cereal grains, and breads, as well as many vegetables and fruits from column A and D, are called complex-carbohydrate foods. Diets that contain ample complex carbohydrates make good nutritional sense. Ounce per ounce, carbohydrates contain less than half the calories of fats. And complex carbohydrates are better for you than simple carbohydrates like sugars, which provide calories but little else in the way of nutritional value. Complex carbohydrates are also a natural source of dietary fiber.

Portion sizes of meat, fish, and poultry need no modification to be compatible with levels of protein generally recommended by nutritionists. Of course during maintenance, you do not have to be so precise about portion sizes of main-course items. An extra-large helping of meat, fish, or poultry every so often is fine. The key is moderation and keeping portion sizes at the appropriate level most of the time.

Off Day meals are fairly low in fat. The low-fat cooking methods used during the Two-Day Diet can become the standard way you prepare foods in the future because you will by now have learned how good vegetables taste steamed or stir-fried in a little oil, how well chicken tastes skinned, seared in a hot skillet, and then simmered in stock with fresh seasonings and vegetables, and how moist and delicious fish can be brushed with oil, sprinkled with lemon, then broiled. The heavy use of butter, margarine, or vegetable oil in cooking is counterproductive to long-term maintenance. So is the use of rich gravies and creamy sauces. You don't have to ban these foods. In fact, you may have been eating them regularly in small amounts as cravers during Off Days. Once again, the key is moderation and common sense.

We have already discussed limiting cholesterol consumption during the Two-Day Diet. Eggs, red meat, cheeses, and whole-milk products should all be kept to the sensible and prudent levels on the maintenance program. In general, orient your meals toward fish or poultry main dishes, limit eggs to approximately three per week, and stick to the low-fat milk, yogurt, and cheeses.

What about cravers? Items from the cravers list and similar kinds of rich, high-calorie foods fit perfectly well into a program of weight maintenance. Limit yourself to about two cravers per day. However, if a special occasion comes along, feel free to indulge without guilt—have an excellent sauce or cream-based soup in a restaurant, a wonderful dessert at a dinner party. Life would be dull without them. Do try to minimize sugary cravers in your diet. Cookies, candy bars, and cakes all have limited nutritional value and tend to increase appetite and hunger. Fresh fruits like apples, oranges, and bananas make far better choices as between-meal snacks. And remember if a particular craver is your Achilles stomach, it is best to keep it out of the house to prevent an uncontrollable binge.

Vitamin and mineral supplementation is particularly important during the initial rapid weight-loss phase of the Two-Day Diet. During maintenance, calories are less restricted and the need for nutrient supplementation is less. Most people will fully achieve their minimal daily requirements for vitamins and minerals during their maintenance period. However, some people, particularly women, who need generous levels of calcium and iron in their diets, may not satisfy all their vitamin and mineral needs. As indicated in Chapter 11, women should get into the habit of choosing foods high in calcium and iron. If you believe you have a need for supplementation, a daily multivitamin/mineral tablet is a reasonable insurance against dietary deficiencies.

You may have noticed two omissions in the discussion of weight maintenance. First, we haven't told you precisely how far to increase portion sizes over and above the usual Off Day portion sizes. Second, we haven't mentioned the number of calories you should aim to consume daily. Long-term weight maintenance is not a calorie-counting exercise. People should not be expected to measure portion sizes for the rest of their lives. These are simply not practical approaches, and they are certainly not pleasant. Weight maintenance must be tailored to the needs of each individual. Some fortunate people will find it relatively easy to maintain their weight loss and may be able to take a fairly casual approach to calorie control. Others will find it difficult to maintain their weight loss and may have to pay close attention to portion sizes.

Will you find it easy or hard to keep weight off? The answer depends on a number of factors, including the length of time you have been overweight, your genetic predisposition, and how diligently you have been following your exercise program. The only way to know for certain is to enter the maintenance period and monitor yourself closely. Don't be afraid of the scales. Weigh yourself frequently, at least once per week. If you catch your weight rising, take immediate action. Analyze your eating habits during maintenance. How far do they deviate from conventional Off Day meals? Have you vastly increased portion sizes of starches, fruits, and vegetables? Are you losing control at restaurants or lunches at work? Have you stopped exercising? Candidly answer these questions and aggressively tackle problem areas. You have the knowledge and ability to achieve long-term weight control.

EXERCISE AND WEIGHT MAINTENANCE

We cannot say this too strongly: Exercise is the key to successful long-term maintenance. The Two-Day Diet exercise program helps you become leaner and raises your metabolic rate. The maintenance-period exercise program will help keep you lean and keep your metabolic rate geared up. Your overall fitness level is greatly improved during the initial phases of the Two-Day Diet. The maintenance-period exercise plan will further increase your new level of fitness. The fitter you are, the more you can eat without weight regain. It's as simple as that. You can be highly optimistic about maintaining your new weight if you are committed to regular physical activity. Without exercise, weight maintenance would become a grind: You would probably find it difficult to increase food consumption much beyond a typical Off Day level. That would make you a chronic dieter. We want you to become a weight maintainer—and that's considerably easier.

One of the great things about fitness is that once you've got it, it's relatively easy to keep it. Let's reflect on your path to fitness on the Two-Day Diet. During the initial stage of the diet, you engage in light exercise for at least five days per week for at least thirty minutes a session. Light exercise raises your heartbeat to a level of 60 to 70 percent of its maximum rate and promotes burning of fat stores by working muscles. Most people will take three weeks or longer to reach their target weight-loss goal. By the time you reach your target, you will have gone a long way toward the attainment of cardiovascular fitness. During the two-week metabolic adjustment period, you engage in moderate exercise for at least five days per week for at least thirty minutes a session. Moderate exercise raises your heart rate to a level of 70 to 85 percent of maximum. It further increases your fitness and helps you get through the critical transition from dieting to maintaining. The exercise program for weight maintenance will take less of your time and will be easier to fit into your schedule:

All You Need to Do Is Engage in Moderate Exercise at Least Three Times a Week for at Least Twenty Minutes a Session

Aim to keep your heart rate in the 70 to 85 percent range of your age-predicted maximum throughout the session. The target heart-rate chart on page 185 for the metabolic adjustment period may also be used for the maintenance period. Choose an activity that works well for you. By this point, you should have settled on those exercises that fit your temperament and schedule. Continue to include five-minute warm-up and cool-down activities before and after your exercise session. The group of seven stretch-and-tone exercises may also be carried out indefinitely. It is important to space your exercise sessions evenly throughout the week—for example, Monday, Wednesday, Saturday or Tuesday, Thursday, Sunday. Try not to let more than two days elapse between workouts. Keep these sessions varied and keep them fun. If one type of activity gets stale, try something else. Bring exercise gear with you on business trips, exercise with friends, consider joining a health club.

At a certain point, which will come sooner than you might imagine, something remarkable will happen to you. You won't need to push yourself to exercise. You won't need a cheerleader to get you off the sofa and into your athletic shoes. You will *want* to exercise. It will sneak up on you like an addiction, except that this kind of addiction is good for you. When this happens and moderate exercise becomes a pleasurable part of your weekly routine, you will have lost something permanently from your life—*the need to ever diet again*.

SOME FINAL WORDS

Rapid, safe weight loss followed by long-term weight maintenance. Does this sound like an impossible goal for you? It's not. The unique metabolic and motivational approach of the Two-Day Diet puts this goal well within your reach. Now that you've read the book, you know that this is no ordinary diet, certainly not a fad diet. It is based on sound scientific principles but represents a completely new concept in dieting. Start soon, and don't worry about failing. After all, anyone can stay on a diet for two days.

Appendix I:

Determining Your Weight-Loss Goal

Instructions

This chart, developed by obesity specialist George Bray, may be used to approximate your personal weight-loss goal. All you need to know is your current weight without clothes, in pounds or kilograms, and your height without shoes, in inches or centimeters. Hold one end of a ruler or straight edge at the point on the chart that indicates your weight. Then pivot the ruler so that it rests at the correct point in the height chart. Draw a line connecting the two points. The place where this line intersects with the center scale is your "body mass index" (weight divided by height, squared). By the zones marked on either side of this index scale, you can determine if you are obese, overweight, or in the acceptable zone.

To find out roughly how much weight you should lose, keep the edge of the ruler or straight edge on your height and move it to the point on the body-mass index scale where it falls just within the upper limit of the acceptable range. Draw a straight line extending through the weight scale.

The difference between your current weight and acceptable
weight is an estimate of a sensible weight-loss goal.

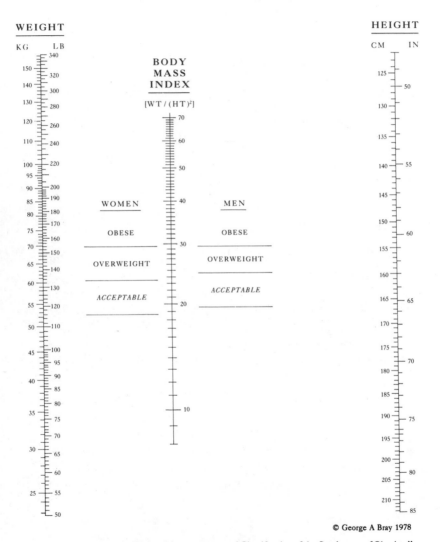

© George A Bray 1978

Bray, George A.: "Definition, Measurement, and Classification of the Syndromes of Obesity."
International Journal of Obesity: 99–112, 1978

Two-Day Diet Menu-Planning Charts for Three Weeks

Monday—On Day

Breakfast

☕ _____

_____

_____

_____

☐   ☐   ☐
A   B   C

Lunch

🍴 _____

_____

_____

_____

☐   ☐   ☐
A   B   C

Dinner

🍴 _____

_____

_____

_____

☐   ☐   ☐
A   B   C

Tuesday—On Day

Breakfast

☕ _____

_____

_____

_____

☐   ☐   ☐
A   B   C

Lunch

🍴 _____

_____

_____

_____

☐   ☐   ☐
A   B   C

Dinner

🍴 _____

_____

_____

_____

☐   ☐   ☐
A   B   C

Wednesday—Off Day

Breakfast

☐ _____

_____

_____

_____

☐   ☐   ☐
A   B   C

Lunch

_____

_____

_____

_____

☐   ☐   ☐   ☐
A   B   C   D

_____
craver

Dinner

_____

_____

_____

_____

☐   ☐   ☐   ☐
A   B   C   D

_____
craver

Thursday—On Day

Breakfast

☕ _____

_____

_____

_____

☐   ☐   ☐
A   B   C

Lunch

🍴 _____

_____

_____

_____

☐   ☐   ☐
A   B   C

Dinner

🍴 _____

_____

_____

_____

☐   ☐   ☐
A   B   C

Friday—On Day

Breakfast

☕ _____

_____

_____

_____

☐   ☐   ☐
A   B   C

Lunch

🍴 _____

_____

_____

_____

☐   ☐   ☐
A   B   C

Dinner

🍴 _____

_____

_____

_____

☐   ☐   ☐
A   B   C

Saturday—Off Day

Breakfast

☕ _____

_____

_____

_____

☐   ☐   ☐
A   B   C

Lunch

🍴 _____

_____

_____

_____

☐   ☐   ☐   ☐
A   B   C   D

_____
craver

Dinner

🍴 _____

_____

_____

_____

☐   ☐   ☐   ☐
A   B   C   D

_____
craver

Sunday—Off Day

Breakfast

☕ _____

_____

_____

_____

☐ ☐ ☐
A B C

Lunch

🍴 _____

_____

_____

_____

_____

☐ ☐ ☐ ☐
A B C D

_____
craver

Dinner

🍴 _____

_____

_____

_____

_____

☐ ☐ ☐ ☐
A B C D

_____
craver

Monday—On Day

Breakfast

☕ _____

_____

_____

_____

☐   ☐   ☐
A   B   C

Lunch

🍴 _____

_____

_____

_____

☐   ☐   ☐
A   B   C

Dinner

🍴 _____

_____

_____

_____

☐   ☐   ☐
A   B   C

Tuesday—On Day

Breakfast

_____

_____

_____

_____

☐   ☐   ☐
A   B   C

Lunch

_____

_____

_____

_____

☐   ☐   ☐
A   B   C

Dinner

_____

_____

_____

_____

☐   ☐   ☐
A   B   C

Wednesday—Off Day

Breakfast

_____

_____

_____

_____

☐   ☐   ☐
A   B   C

Lunch

_____

_____

_____

_____

_____

☐   ☐   ☐   ☐
A   B   C   D

_____
craver

Dinner

_____

_____

_____

_____

_____

☐   ☐   ☐   ☐
A   B   C   D

_____
craver

Thursday—On Day

Breakfast

☐ A ☐ B ☐ C

Lunch

☐ A ☐ B ☐ C

Dinner

☐ A ☐ B ☐ C

Friday—On Day

Breakfast

☕ _____

_____

_____

_____

☐ ☐ ☐
A   B   C

Lunch

🍴 _____

_____

_____

_____

☐ ☐ ☐
A   B   C

Dinner

🍴 _____

_____

_____

_____

☐ ☐ ☐
A   B   C

Saturday—Off Day

☕ *Breakfast*
_____

_____

_____

_____

☐ ☐ ☐
A   B   C

🍴 *Lunch*
_____

_____

_____

_____

☐ ☐ ☐ ☐
A   B   C   D

_____
craver

🍴 *Dinner*
_____

_____

_____

_____

☐ ☐ ☐ ☐
A   B   C   D

_____
craver

Sunday—Off Day

Breakfast

_____

_____

_____

_____

☐ ☐ ☐
A   B   C

Lunch

_____

_____

_____

_____

_____

☐ ☐ ☐ ☐
A   B   C   D

_____
craver

Dinner

_____

_____

_____

_____

_____

☐ ☐ ☐ ☐
A   B   C   D

_____
craver

Monday—On Day

Breakfast

A B C

Lunch

A B C

Dinner

A B C

Tuesday—On Day

Breakfast

☕

☐   ☐   ☐
A   B   C

Lunch

🍴

☐   ☐   ☐
A   B   C

Dinner

✖

☐   ☐   ☐
A   B   C

Wednesday—Off Day

Breakfast

☕ _____

_____

_____

_____

☐ ☐ ☐
A   B   C

Lunch

🍴 _____

_____

_____

_____

☐ ☐ ☐ ☐
A   B   C   D

_____
craver

Dinner

🍴 _____

_____

_____

_____

☐ ☐ ☐ ☐
A   B   C   D

_____
craver

Thursday—On Day

Breakfast

☐ A ☐ B ☐ C

Lunch

☐ A ☐ B ☐ C

Dinner

☐ A ☐ B ☐ C

Friday—On Day

Breakfast

_____

_____

_____

_____

☐ ☐ ☐
A   B   C

Lunch

_____

_____

_____

_____

☐ ☐ ☐
A   B   C

Dinner

_____

_____

_____

_____

☐ ☐ ☐
A   B   C

Saturday—Off Day

Breakfast

☐ ☐ ☐
A   B   C

Lunch

☐ ☐ ☐ ☐
A   B   C   D

craver

Dinner

☐ ☐ ☐ ☐
A   B   C   D

craver

Sunday—Off Day

Breakfast

☕ _____

_____

_____

_____

☐　☐　☐
A　B　C

Lunch

🍴 _____

_____

_____

_____

_____

☐　☐　☐　☐
A　B　C　D

_____
craver

Dinner

🍴 _____

_____

_____

_____

_____

☐　☐　☐　☐
A　B　C　D

_____
craver

Subject Index

Abdominal curl-up (stretch and tone exercise), 162
Achilles stomach, 78
Aerobics, 156
Airline food, adapting, 150
Alcohol, 26–27
  fat storage and, 27
  ketosis and, 31
Alcoholic beverages for Off Days, 72
Antihypertensive medications, 174
Appetite suppression
  LCHP diets and, 32
  during On Days, 149
Arthritis, 176
Artificial sweeteners, 74

Bacon, 74, 85
Baking, 62, 149
Bananas, 60
Beer for Off Days, 72
Behavioral approaches to obesity treatment, 5–6
Blood fats (lipids), elevated, 174–75
Blood sugar, elevated, 173
Body composition, 22–27
  alcohol and, 26–27
  carbohydrate storage, 23–24, 30
  fat storage, 24–25
  protein storage, 25–26
Body-fat content, 21–22
Body mass index, 195
Body weight, 19–22

Bouillon, 64
Breads, 23, 62, 75
  on Off Days, 74
  whole wheat, 75
Breakfast
  fasted-state metabolism and, 28–29
  importance of, 149
  for Off days, 74
    Master Menu, 67
    recipes for breakfast dishes, 145–46
    sample menus, 90, 93, 94, 97, 100, 101, 104, 107, 108
  for On Days, 60–61
    Master Menu, 56
    recipes for breakfast dishes, 127–28
    sample menus, 88, 89, 91, 92, 95, 96, 98, 99, 105, 106
Breast-feeding mothers, 43
  nutritional requirements needed for, 170–71
Broiling, 62, 85
Brown rice, 75
Brunch, 151–52
Business meals, 151, 152
Butter, 24, 75

Cafeteria dining, 48, 150
Calcium, 33, 63
  On Days breakfast and, 61
  requirements for women, 50, 171–72

Calf stretch (stretch and tone exercise), 162, 165–66
Calories
  alcohol and, 26–27
  daily content of Off Days menus, 46
  daily content of On Days menus, 45
  stored in carbohydrates, 23
  stored in fats, 24–25
  stored in proteins, 26
Canned fruit, 63
Canned vegetables, 62
Carbohydrates, 22, 23–24, 27
  dieting and, 30
  during maintenance period, 189–90
  Off Days and, 46
  On Days and, 45, 60
Cardiovascular disease, hypertension and, 173
Celery, 63
Cellulose, 23
Cereals, 23, 74
  high-bran, 50, 177
Cheating on diets, 15–16
Cheese, 60–61, 62, 74
Chicken, 61
  portion sizes for, 52
Children, 43
  nondieting, 148–49
Cholesterol
  elevated, 174–75
  limitations on, 50
  during maintenance period, 190
Club soda, 64
Cocktails for Off Days, 72
Coffee, 64
Condiments, 64
  for Off Days menus, 72
Cooked vegetables, 61, 62
Cookies, 77
Cottage cheese, 60–61, 62
Cravers
  during maintenance period, 190–91

  during metabolic adjustment period, 184
  for Off Days, 72, 76–78
Cycling, 156

Dairy foods, 60–61, 62, 63, 76
  as cravers for Off Days, 72
  low-fat, 75
  for women, 50
Desserts for Off Days, 77
Diabetes, 43, 172–73
  ketosis and, 31
Dieting with a partner, 41
Diet soda, 64
Dinners
  for Off Days, 74–76
    Master Menu (for men), 70
    Master Menu (for women), 68–69, 71
    sample menus, 90, 93, 94, 97, 100, 101, 104, 107, 108
  for On Days, 61–63
    Master Menu (for men and women), 57–58
    sample menus, 88, 89, 91, 92, 95, 96, 98, 99, 105, 106
Diverticular disease, 177
Dry cereals, 74

Eating out, Master Menu flexibility and, 48, 151–53
Eggs, 50, 60, 85
  for Off Days breakfasts, 74
  protein storage and, 25
  restricting consumption of, 175, 189
Elbow-knee crunch (stretch and tone execise), 162, 163
Elevated blood fats (lipids), 174–75
Elevated blood sugar, 173
Elevated cholesterol, 174–75
Employee cafeteria, 48, 150
Ethnic restaurants, 153
Exercise, metabolism and, 33–39

Exercise program, 53, 154–68
  attaining weight-loss goal, 168
  cool down phase, 149, 161
  defeating the repletion reaction
    and, 180–81, 184
  features of, 155
  light exercise period, 158, 160
  long-term weight maintenance
    and, 168, 192–94
  during metabolic adjustment
    period, 184–86
  on Off Days, 79
  for people with arthritis, 176
  for people with heart disease,
    175–76
  preferred activities for, 156
  rules for starting, 51
  set-point theory and, 7
  stretch and tone exercises, 159,
    161–66
  structure of, 158–59
  tracking one's progress, 166–68
  warming-up phase, 158, 159

Failure of traditional diet plans,
    3–6, 10–17
Family life, 148–49
Fasted-stated metabolism
  dieting and, 29–30
  fed-state metabolism versus,
    28–29
Fast-food items, 75
Fat(s), 22, 24–25, 27
  body content, 21–22
  burning of, 35–37
    On Days, 45–46
  carbohydrates and, 24
  fasted-state metabolism and,
    29
  ketones and, 31
  during maintenance period,
    190
  Off Days and, 46
  set-point theory and, 7
Fatty acids, 24, 26, 27
Fed-state metabolism, fasted-
  state metabolism versus,
    28–29
Fiber source, 50, 177
Finger food, avoiding, 151
Fish, 62, 84
  portion sizes for, 52
  protein storage and, 25
Frozen foods, 75
Frozen vegetables, 61, 62
Fruit, 60, 63
  during maintenance period,
    189
Fruit juices, 60
Fruit yogurt, 77

Glucose, 23, 24, 26, 27
  production of, 29
Glycogen, 23–24, 35
  fasted-state metabolism and,
    28–29
Grapefruit, 60
Grilling, 62
Grocery shopping, 49

Hamburgers, 75
  portion sizes for, 52
Hamstring stretch (stretch and
    tone exercise), 162, 165
Heart disease, 43, 175–76
Heart rates
  for light exercise, 158
  for moderate exercise, 185
Height-weight tables, 19, 20–21
High blood pressure, 43, 173–74
High-bran cereals, 50, 177
High-fiber diets for intestinal dis-
    orders, 177
Hormones, 25
  transition from fed-state to
    fasted-state and, 28
Hydrostatic weighing (underwater
    weighing) in assessing
    body-fat content, 21
Hypertension (elevated blood
    pressure), 173–74

Ice cream, 78
Illness and injuries, On Days–Off
    Days regime and, 50
Insulin hormone, 28, 172, 173
    LCHP diets and, 31
Intestinal disorders, 177
Invisible fat, 24
Iron requirements for women,
    171
Irregular heartbeat, 33
Irritable colitis, 177

Jogging, 156
Juvenile-onset diabetes, 172

Ketchup, 64
Ketones, 31
Ketosis, 31
    on LCHP diets, 33
    On Days and, 46, 65
Kidney problems, 43

Lettuce, 61,63
Life-styles, 147–53
    family life, 148–49
    social engagements, 151–53
    traditional diet plans and, 17
    the workplace, 149–50
Light (low-intensity) exercise,
    53, 157–58, 160
    fat burning and, 35–37
    metabolism and, 34–35
    target heart rates for, 158
Lipids (blood fats), elevated,
    174–75
Liver, the
    carbohydrate storage and, 24
    protein storage and, 26
Low-calorie bread, 60
Low-calorie salad dressings, 63–
    64, 76
Low-carbohydrate, high-protein
    (LCHP) diets, 30–33
    safety of, 32–33
Lower back stretch (stretch and
    tone exercise), 162, 163
Low-fat milk, 63
Lunches

for Off Days, 74–76
    Master Menu (for men), 70
    Master Menu (for women),
    68–69, 71
    sample menus, 90, 93, 94,
    97, 100, 101, 104, 107,
    108
for On Days, 61–63
    Master Menu (for men and
    women), 57–58
    sample menus, 88, 89, 91,
    92, 95, 96, 98, 99, 105,
    106
at the workplace, 149–50

Maintenance period, 54, 187–194
    guidelines for diet program in
    preparation for, 182–84
    long-term weight maintenance
    diet program and, 188–92
    exercise program and, 168,
    192–94
Margarine, 24
Master Menus, 47–48, 49, 80–
    108
    dining in restaurants, cafete-
    rias, the workplace and,
    48, 150, 151, 152
    food preparation techniques
    for, 81–86
    high-calcium selections from,
    172
    low-cholesterol selections from,
    175
    menu planning, 86–87
    for Odd Days
        breakfasts, 67
        as foundation of mainte-
        nance period, 189–92
        lunches/dinners (for men),
        70
        lunches/dinners (for women),
        68–69, 71
        metabolic adjustment period
        and, 182–84
    for On Days
        breakfasts, 56

lunches/dinners (for men and women), 57–58
sample menus
Off Days (week one), 90, 93–94
Off Days (week two), 97, 100–101
Off Days (week three), 104, 107–8
On Days (week one), 88–89, 91–92
On Days (week two), 95–96, 98–99
On Days (week three), 102–3, 105–6
Maturity-onset diabetes, 172–73
Mayonnaise, 77
Meats, 25, 50, 62, 75, 85
portion sizes for, 52
Medical clearance for Two-Day Diet, 43
Men, daily calorie requirements for, 23
Menu-planning aids, see Master Menus
Menu-planning charts, 197–218
Metabolic adjustment period, 54, 181–86
diet component of, 182–84
exercise component of, 168, 184–86
Metabolic rate
for fat and thin people, 7
set-point theory and, 6–7
Metabolism, 9, 18–39
body composition and, 22–27
body weight and, 19–22
dieting and fasting and, 29–30
exercise and, 33–39
as fuel burning and fuel storage, 18–19
LCHP diets and, 30–33
Off Days and, 46–47
On Days and, 45–46
repletion reaction and, 179–80
transition from fed-state to fasted-state, 28–29
Microwave meals, 75

Milk, 62, 63, 76
Mineral water, 64
Moderate exercise
during long-term weight maintenance period, 193–94
target heart rates for, 185
Monday, starting the Two-Day Diet on, 49
Motivation, 9, 10–17
importance of maintaining life style, 17
incentives and rewards, 13
On Days–Off Days pattern and, 44–45, 47
practicality of the Two-Day Diet plan, 14–15
variety of foods offered, 13–14
Multivitamin/mineral supplement, 46, 50, 65, 79
during maintenance period, 191
for women, 171
Muscle
fasted-state metabolism and, 29
LCHP diets and, 31
muscular development, 36
protein storage and, 25–26

Natural food cravings, 15
Nondieting family members, 148–49
NutraSweet, 64
Nutritional requirements for women, see Women, nutritional requirements for

Oat-bran morning health drink, 74
Off Days, 44–45, 46–47, 66–79
breakfasts for, 74
Master Menu, 67
cravers for, 72, 76–78
do's and don'ts for, 79
eating at the workplace, 149–50
family life and, 148–49
lunches/dinners for, 74–76

Off Days (cont'd)
  Master Menu (for men), 70
  Master Menu (for women),
    68–69, 71
  Master Menus for, 47–48
  as foundation of mainte-
    nance period, 189–92
  metabolic adjustment period
    and, 182–84
  sample menus (week one),
    90, 93–94
  sample menus (week two),
    97, 100–101
  sample menus (week three),
    104, 107–8
  menu planning charts (for
    three weeks), 200, 203–4,
    207, 210–11, 214, 217–18
  recipes for, 48, 129–46
  restaurant dining during, 153
  social engagements during,
    151–53
  unlimited foods during, 73, 76
Office snacks on Off Days, 149
On Days, 44–46, 55–65
  breakfasts for, 60–61
    Master Menu, 56
  do's and don'ts for, 64–65
  eating at the workplace and,
    149–50
  family life and, 148–49
  lunches/dinners for, 61–63
    Master Menu (for men and
    women), 57–58
  Master Menus for, 47–48
  sample menus (week one),
    88–89, 91–92
  sample menus (week two),
    95–96, 98–99
  sample menus (week three),
    102–3, 105–6
  menu-planning charts (for
    three weeks), 198–99,
    201–2, 205–6, 208–9,
    212–13, 215–16
  natural appetite suppression
    during, 149
  recipes for, 48, 111–28

restaurant dining during, 153
social engagements during,
  151, 152–53
unlimited foods during, 59,
  63–64
Open-face sandwiches, 63
Osteoarthritis, 176
Osteoporosis, 171–72

Pan broiling meat, 85
Parties, 151
Partners, dieting with, 41
Pasta, 23, 75
Peanut butter, 74
People who should not partici-
  pate in the Two-Day
  Diet, 43
Pizza, 75
Portion sizes, 51–52
Potatoes, 23, 75
Poultry, 62
  portion sizes for, 52
Pregnant women, 43
  nutritional requirements for,
    170–71
Prescription medications, 43
Proteins, 22, 25–26, 27
  LCHP diets and, 32–33
  Off Days and, 46
  On Days and, 45
  breakfasts, 60–61
Pulse, taking one's own, 158
Push-ups (stretch and tone exer-
  cise), 162, 164

Recipes, 48, 49, 109–46
  how to use, 110–11
  for Off Days, 48, 129–46
  for On Days, 48, 111–28
  See also Recipe Index
Repletion reaction, 54, 179–80
  defeating, 180–88
  exercise program and, 184
Restaurant dining, 48, 150, 151,
  152, 153
Rice, 75
Rowing machine, 156
Rules for starting and following
  the Two-Day Diet, 48–51

Saccharin, 64
Salad greens, 61, 63
Salad oil, 24
Salads, 61–62
    as unlimited foods, 63–64
Salt, 64
Salt-restricted diet, 64
Salty foods during metabolic ad-
        justment period, 183
Sandwiches, open-face, 63
Snacks
    for nondieting children, 149
    for Off Days, 72, 77
Set-point theory, 6–7, 179
Shellfish, 62
Shopping for groceries, 49
Social engagements, 48, 151–53
Sour cream, 77
Spinach, 61, 63
Starches, 23
Steaming fish, 84
Steaming vegetables, 81–82
Stir-frying, 82
Stretch and tone exercises, 159,
        161–66
Sugars, 23
Sugary cravers
    during maintenance period, 191
    during metabolic adjustment
        period, 184
Sunday brunch, 151–52
Sweetened cereals, 74
Sweeteners, artificial, 74
Sweets for Off Days, 72
Swimming, 156, 176

Taste change as On Days possi-
        bility, 65
Tea, 64
Teenagers, 43
Thin people, set-point theory
        and, 7
Tomatoes, 61
Traditional diets, failure of, 3–6,
        10–17
Traveling, adapting meals for,
        150
Tuna, 61, 63, 75

Unbalanced diets, 30–32
Unlimited foods, 59, 63–64, 73,
        76
Upper back and side stretch
        (stretch and tone exer-
        cise), 162, 164–65

Vegetable oils, 24
Vegetables, 50, 61–62, 75, 81–82
    during maintenance period,
        189
Visible fat, 24

Walking, 156
Water
    on Off Days, 79
    on On Days, 46, 64
Weight control, metabolism and,
        18–19
Weight loss, 41–42
    during Off Days, 47
Weight loss goal
    attaining, 168
    charting progress, 167
    establishing, 42–43, 195–96
    metabolic adjustment period
        and, 178, 180, 182
Weight maintenance, long-term
    diet program and, 188–92
    exercise program and, 168,
        192–94
Whole wheat bread, 75
Wine for Off Days, 72
Women, 170–72
    daily calorie requirements for,
        23
    nutritional requirements for
        calcium, 50, 171–72
        iron, 171
        during pregnancy and while
            breast-feeding, 170–71
Workplace, 149–50

Yogurt, 60, 74
    fruit, 77

Recipe Index

Almonds, baked fish and, 133
Ambrosia, 140–41
Apple(s)
cinnamon, crêpes, 142
torte, 144

Bacon, preparation technique for, 85
Banana(s)
frappe, 127
morning health drink, 145
nut bread, 143–44
Beverages
banana frappe, 127
morning health drink, 145
strawberry yogurt shake, 128
Breads, 23, 62
banana nut, 143–44
Broccoli and cauliflower, stir-fried, 139

Cake, cheese, 142–43
Carrots, lentils and, 138
Cauliflower and broccoli, stir-fried, 139
Cheeseburgers, 121
Cheese cake, 142–43
Chef's salad deluxe, 123–24
Chicken
coq au vin, 129
curried, with rice, 130–31
lemon, 113–14
paprika with yogurt, 130
portion sizes for, 52
preparation techniques for, 83
Provençal, 113
stock, 115
sweet and sour, 114
tarragon, 112
teriyaki, 111–12

Waldorf salad with, 131–32
Chiliburgers, 120
Cinnamon apple crêpes, 142
Coq au vin, 129
Country burgers, 121
Creole sauce, pork chops in, 122
Crêpes
cinnamon apple, 142
ratatouille, 136–38
Curried chicken with rice, 130–31

Desserts
ambrosia, 140–41
apple torte, 144
cheese cake, 142–43
cinnamon apple crêpes, 142
peach Melba, 141
Swiss-style yogurt, 141

Eggplant Parmesan, 136
Eggs
Benedict, 146
preparation techniques for, 85

Fish
baked, and almonds, 133
braised, with julienne vegetables, 132
plaki, 116
portion sizes for, 52
preparation techniques for, 83–84
protein storage and, 25
See also Flounder; Shellfish; Swordfish; Tuna fish
Flounder
portion sizes for, 52
wrapped baked, 115–16

Food preparation techniques, 81–86
cooking with herbs and spices, 86
eggs, 85
fish, 83–84
meat, 84–85
poultry, 83
vegetables, 81–82
Frappe, banana, 127
French toast, 127
Fruit
ambrosia, 140–41
See also names of fruit

Garden pasta salad, 139–40
Garlic, lamb chops with rosemary and, 122–23
Gazpacho, 125–26
Green peppers
hamburgers with mushrooms and, 120
stuffed, 119
Grilling meat, 84–85

Hamburgers
with mushrooms and peppers, 120
other ideas for, 120–21
portion sizes for, 52
preparation techniques for, 84–85
Hawaiian shrimp kebabs, 117
Herbs
cooking with, 86
See also names of herbs

Kebabs, Hawaiian shrimp, 117

Lamb chops
with garlic and rosemary, 122–23
portion sizes for, 52

Lemon chicken, 113–14
Lemon juice as salad dressing, 64
Lentils and carrots, 138
Lobster, portion sizes for, 52
Low-calorie salad dressing, 63–64
Meats, 25, 50, 62
    portion sizes for, 52
    preparation techniques for, 84–85
    See also Hamburgers; Lamb chops; Pork chops; Veal
Melon salad, 126
Morning health drink, 145
Mushrooms
    hamburgers with peppers and, 120
    scallops with tomatoes and, 117–18
    veal with, 121

Oriental vegetables, 125

Pancakes, 145
Paprika, chicken, with yogurt, 130
Parmesan cheese, eggplant with, 136
Pasta, 23
    garden salad with, 139–40
    primavera, 135
    tuna sauce for, 134
Peach Melba, 141
Peppercorns, hamburgers au poivre, 120
Peppers, see Green peppers
Poaching fish, 84
Pork chops
    baked stuffed, 133–34
    in Creole sauce, 122
    portion sizes for, 52
Portion sizes for food, 51–52
Poultry, 62
    portion sizes for, 52

preparation techniques for, 83
    See also Chicken
Provençal chicken, 113

Ratatouille, crêpes, 136–38
Rice, curried chicken with, 130–31
Rosemary, lamb chops with garlic and, 122–23

Salad dressing
    low-calorie, 63–64
    vinaigrette, 140
    "vinegarette," 63–64, 124
Salads, 61–62
    chef's, deluxe, 123–24
    garden pasta, 139–40
    melon, 126
    tuna fish, 118
    as unlimited food, 63–64
    Waldorf chicken, 131–32
Sauces
    Creole, 122
    for Off Days menus, 73
    tuna pasta, 134
Scallops
    with mushrooms and tomatoes, 117–18
    portion sizes for, 52
Shake, strawberry yogurt, 128
Shellfish, 62
    See also Scallops; Shrimp
Shrimp
    kebabs, Hawaiian, 117
    portion sizes for, 52
Soup
    chicken stock, 115
    gazpacho, 125–26
Spices, 64
    cooking with, 86
    See also names of spices
Steaming fish, 84
Steaming vegetables, 81–82
Stir-fried (stir-frying)
    broccoli and cauliflower, 139

vegetables, 82
Stock, chicken, 115
Strawberry yogurt shake, 128
Sweet and sour chicken, 114
Swiss-style yogurt, 141
Swordfish, portion sizes for, 52

Tarragon chicken, 112
Teriyaki chicken, 111–12
Toast, French, 127
Tomatoes
    scallops with mushrooms and, 117–18
    zucchini and, 123–24
Torte, apple, 144
Tuna fish, 63
    pasta sauce, 134
    salad, 118

Veal with mushrooms, 121
Vegetables, 50, 61–62
    crêpes ratatouille, 136–38
    garden pasta salad, 139–40
    julienne, braised fish with, 132
    Oriental, 125
    pasta primavera, 135
    preparation techniques for, 81–82
    See also names of vegetables
Vinaigrette dressing, 140
"Vinegarette" dressing, 63–64, 124

Waldorf chicken salad, 131–32
Wine for cooking, 83

Yogurt
    chicken paprika with, 130
    strawberry shake, 128
    Swiss-style, 141

Zucchini and tomatoes, 123–24

About the Authors

TESSA COOPER has a master's degree in nutrition from Tufts University and a degree in physical education from Northeastern University.

DR. GLENN COOPER is a Harvard-trained physician who is a specialist in internal medicine.